Joanna Blythman is Britain's leading investigative food journalist and an influential commentator on the British scene, as well as being the mother of two young children. She has won two prestigious Glenfiddich awards for her writing as well as the Caroline Walker Media Award for 'Improving the Nation's Health by means of Good Food'. She writes for the *Guardian* newspaper, and is a regular contributor to *Scotland on Sunday*, several magazines and Radio 4's *The Food Programme*.

The Food We Eat

The Food We Eat

The book you cannot afford to ignore

JOANNA BLYTHMAN

MICHAEL JOSEPH
LONDON

MICHAEL JOSEPH LTD

Published by the Penguin Group
27 Wrights Lane, London W8 5TZ
Viking Penguin Inc., 375 Hudson Street, New York, New York 10014, USA
Penguin Books Australia Ltd, Ringwood, Victoria, Australia
Penguin Books Canada Ltd, 10 Alcorn Avenue, Toronto, Ontario, Canada M4V 3B2
Penguin Books (NZ) Ltd, 182–190 Wairau Road, Auckland 10, New Zealand

Penguin Books Ltd, Registered Offices: Harmondsworth, Middlesex, England

First published 1996
10 9 8 7 6 5 4 3

Typeset in 10.5/12.75pt Monophoto Bembo.
Printed in England by Clays Ltd, St Ives plc

A CIP catalogue record for this book is available from the British Library

ISBN 0 7181 3912 7

Contents

Acknowledgements

The author would like to acknowledge the time, effort and input of all the following people, who were generous enough to share their specialist knowledge and advise, check and comment on the text.

Lynda Brown, Martin Cottingham, Sue Dibb, Nicola Fletcher, Charles Franchina, Roy Haycock, Randolph Hodgson, Patrick Holden, John Humphries, Vivien Jawett, Robin Jenkins, Richard Lacey, Diane Lamb, Monica Lavery, John Lister, Tim Lobstein, Sally and John McKenna, Charlotte Mitchell, Martin Pitt, Alan Porter, Brian Scott, Peter Segger, Peter Stevenson, Andrew Whitley, Antony Wild.

A special thank you to my editor, Louise Haines, for coming to me with the idea for this book in the first place and for her constant support thereafter.

This book is written for my daughters – Amy
and Zoe – that they might grow up as part of a generation
that understands food quality and delights
in the pleasure of eating

Introduction

This book is about food quality, and how to recognise good food when you see it, be it a piece of cheese, a leg of lamb, a melon, a packet of coffee or a bar of chocolate. The food we eat these days has never been more diverse, more sophisticated or more difficult to judge. Life used to be a lot simpler. Fruits and vegetables had seasons, hens ran around in farmyards, cows were out to grass, salmon was wild – an early summer treat – and bread was made to time-honoured principles.

Nowadays, seasons have become relatively meaningless, since you can buy raspberries at Christmas and northern European peppers in January. Most of our egg-laying hens spend their lives in batteries. Many of our cows have been transformed into milk machines who live indoors eating concentrated feedstuffs. Nearly all salmon is farmed, and traditional breadmaking has been largely superseded by push-button bread made in vast industrial plants.

There's a growing polarisation in the type of food we eat. The good news here is the return to sound traditional principles of good animal husbandry and careful food production, which manifests itself in the growing number of producers, many organic, who are rediscovering tried-and-tested breeds of animals, flavoursome varieties of fruit and vegetables, and food made with artisan skills.

However, while the motivated shopper fills the trolley with these delights, our shelves are laden with both the products of intensive farming and heavily processed foods whose raw ingredients have been downgraded and compromised in a way that owes more to the laboratory than the kitchen. Genetic engineering can now come up with increasingly outlandish constructions which make the old food colourings and additives seem like child's play. Slowly but surely, gene technology is finding applications in our everyday foodstuffs.

And yet the average shopper takes only a couple of seconds to scan a food label, often buying on trust or out of habit, without much idea of the true quality of the food on offer or the methods by which it is produced. The aware and concerned consumer scrutinises the labels with increasing mistrust and rarely finds the answers to the questions raised.

What this book aims to do is simplify that task a little by putting through their paces all the foods we routinely buy. It looks at how each one matches up to the standards that modern consumers are increasingly demanding – safe, high-quality, wholesome and nutritious food produced with respect for animals, workers in the food industry and the environment. The aim is to empower the interested consumer with the necessary background information so that she or he can make an informed, positive choice from the sometimes baffling array of foods on sale.

As things stand, most of us are inadequately equipped for that task. Over the last 50 years world food production has largely moved away from small-scale localised concerns to global intensive farming – agribusiness. Only a shrinking minority of us has any connection with farmers or growers and the land they work, and so we have little or no insight into the means by which our food is produced.

While the food chain was once a very simple relationship between producer and consumer, it has now become big business. There are lots of cogs and wheels in the chain these days, from the large chemical and bio-tech companies who design seeds and manufacture lucrative chemical products to use alongside them, to the elite club of large transnational companies who control food production in important sectors all over the world. Some of these are also the manufacturers who transform raw foods (not usually for the better) into profitable 'value-added' products. Then there is the handful of extremely powerful supermarket chains, who by virtue of market strength can very nearly dictate the terms on which our food is grown.

Knowledge is power. My hope in writing this book is that by becoming better informed about the way in which our food is produced we can slightly redress the balance of power in favour of the consumer. By dint of our collective buying clout, we can be tremendously influential in demanding high-quality food and changing for the better the future direction of food production.

And what direction should it take? An underlying theme in this book is supporting organic farming whenever and wherever you can. This is because organic farming is the only coherent, regulated alternative form of agriculture capable of satisfying the consumer's demand for natural, wholesome food, as well as finding solutions to environmental problems that are becoming ever more pressing.

Organic food is currently what is known as a 'niche market'. But it could become mainstream with a change at European level in the way that financial support is given to agriculture. More organic food would become available, at prices that everyone could afford. In the meantime, by buying organic when we can, we force that issue higher up the political agenda.

Not everything you read in these pages will leave you feeling comforted. Certain aspects of the British food supply are very unsavoury and it would be dishonest to skim over them however uncomfortable they might make us feel. Furthermore, if your first priority about food is price, you should know now that if you follow the advice in this book you may have to pay more than you currently do for some foods. But you will be receiving far better value for money, you may well find your health improves, and you can make up the shortfall by striking some other foods off your list. It's up to you to decide which ones!

The price that most people without chronic financial problems are prepared to pay for food is largely arbitrary and not particularly consistent. Many British shoppers don't think twice about buying elaborately packaged, manufactured processed foods that are actually extremely expensive, yet they will baulk at paying a modest percentage more for better-quality raw ingredients. So many of us could eat better food for the same financial outlay simply by adjusting our priorities.

The compensation for more thoughtful food shopping is obvious. The consequences of the UK's love affair with cheap food can be seen all around us, in items like spindly, tasteless chickens, bland Golden Delicious apples, watery tomatoes and breads of such staggering uniformity and absence of character that they are hardly worth eating. They're cheap, certainly. But where's the pleasure? And given the hidden cost to our health, the environment and animal welfare, not forgetting the toll taken by the soulless, dehumanising jobs created by modern methods of food production, are these foods really so cheap after all?

The fact is that by demanding cheap food rather than good food we put producers under impossible pressure which can only diminish quality. What we need to develop now is the notion of value for money. Price is something that should reflect the integrity of ingredients and the skill and care with which the food was made, reared, caught or grown. Viewed in this way, the foods recommended in this book make good financial sense. Whatever the size of your wallet and whatever category of food you're looking at – be it bananas, pork chops, fish fingers or Cheddar cheese – *The Food We Eat* will help you make a better choice.

Fruit and Vegetables

Where to buy

A crucial element of quality food shopping these days is locating a good source for fresh fruit and vegetables. Where's best?

SUPERMARKETS

If you do most of your food shopping in a supermarket it is likely that you'll also use it for fruit and vegetables. Supermarkets often seem to offer a dazzling array which places them in a different league from the corner greengrocer. They have reintroduced traditional varieties of apples, pears and potatoes, new types of lettuce and tomatoes, and a lot more besides to a wider public than ever before. In certain prosperous urban quarters the selection of fruit and vegetables can be quite decent, but branches of the same chain in less metropolitan areas are often disappointingly limited.

There are certain key problems with supermarket retailing of fruit and vegetables. The first is packaging. Although an increasing proportion of produce is sold loose, many supermarket fruit and vegetables are wrapped to within an inch of their lives. This particularly applies to the pricier, and often out-of-season, lines that your local greengrocer is unlikely to offer – nectarines at Christmas, special varieties of pear and so on. Although it is meant to be protective, overwrapping means that we cannot use the vital senses of smell and touch to assess the produce and are more likely to make an expensive bad choice.

Then there is the question of range. Supermarkets offer the illusion of choice by trying to stock all fruits and vegetables all year round, sourced worldwide. In fact, the flavour of most out-of-season produce compares very poorly with that sourced in season. Many imported vegetables, such as mangetout, green beans, baby corn, have become such clichés as to no longer excite us. Look at the supermarket range without this type of produce and the choice is not always as great as it seems.

Another issue is the supermarket espousal of 'exotic' produce, loudly trumpeted as a further indicator of the magnificent choice they offer. But how many people do you know who eat New Zealand horned melon, tamarillos or rambutans every week? What are you meant to do with a stick of sugar cane anyway? Viewed cynically, the exotic range in supermarkets just serves as elaborate window dressing.

For all their buying clout, our large chains are remarkably ponderous and unresponsive institutions. Centralisation of buying and distribution through a small number of handling depots means that local stores are not able to respond to seasonal trends in the way the local greengrocer can. This leads to all sorts of silly contortions, such as Scottish stores selling English strawberries at the peak of the Scottish strawberry season, or supermarkets in the Lake District that do not have any damsons while they are being sold in roadside stalls.

Unhappy about all this? Write a letter – supermarkets cannot treat these lightly because they have to make an effort to find out the necessary information and write back. If you haven't got the time to write a letter, talk to the manager of your local store. But don't expect speedy results. You'll have to put your request in the comments book and then the manager will ask central buying whether they will supply it. If your store isn't on that carefully maintained computerised list of projected consumer demand the answer will most likely be, sorry, we can't supply it. But there's lots of horned melons though…

And what of price? Many consumers choose supermarkets in preference to small shops because they think the food is cheaper. Whether this is true or not when it comes to groceries is debatable. But in the produce section, with the exception of two or three prominent promotional lines, supermarket fruit and vegetables are frighteningly expensive, often significantly more so than at the local greengrocer's.

What are you paying for? There's the maintenance of that elaborate distribution system and much-vaunted cold chain, selection by 'our specialist buyers' and so on. In the case of Marks and Spencer, who have become produce specialists, you can taste the effort; it is up to you whether you are prepared to pay the premium. For the other supermarket chains, the results are not always reliable enough to justify the astonishing mark-up. You'll also be paying for all that packaging, like a rigid, attractively coloured plastic tray to support your four baking potatoes, which are then encased in gift-wrap crinkly cellophane. Once you get the stuff home you'll fill the rubbish bin in a flash. Somebody is paying for all that garbage and that person is you!

LOCAL GREENGROCERS

Local greengrocers got a big shock when supermarkets first started taking fruit and vegetables seriously. Many of them needed it, since they were serving up a lacklustre, conservative selection of withered Golden Delicious apples, anonymous 'white' potatoes and wilting Dutch hothouse lettuce.

Many of these have gone to the wall, and we cannot mourn them. A certain amount of fruit and vegetable retailing has been taken on by open-all-hours convenience stores, who have absolutely no expertise in this area. Pretty crummy they tend to be, too. A small minority of dedicated greengrocers has survived. Most significant centres of population still have a shop – often with a second- or third-generation ethnic influence – that makes a good job of offering reasonably priced produce, bought direct from the market. Competition from supermarkets has forced them to become more sophisticated and adventurous.

If you find a good greengrocer's it will beat the average supermarket hands down on price. The shop may seem tiny but, realistically, the choice of goods you actually want to buy will probably be the same or better than in a supermarket. What you won't get is the 'whatever you want, whenever you want it' selection of the supermarket. That's no great loss.

Paper bags for your spuds so they keep better. A chance to poke around and sniff. The possibility of asking an informed human being whether the Moroccan, Spanish or Corsican clementines taste best. All this makes for a much more satisfactory shopping trip, and the bill should be much smaller too.

DIRECT FROM PRODUCERS

If you have a direct link with a producer you can buy some of the freshest, most interesting seasonal produce around. Sick of being squeezed on price by the supermarkets, fed up with the indifference of our wholesale fruit markets, many British producers are selling direct to the public. Home-delivery schemes and farm shops are springing up all over the UK, most of them run by organic growers. If you want baby asparagus and passion fruit all year round you'll be disappointed, since the selection will be strictly local and seasonal, stronger on vegetables than fruit. Some of these schemes can become tedious, with too many repetitions of the same vegetable week in, week out. However, most are capable of fulfilling your basic requirements – carrots, potatoes, onions and so on. The best ones offer a stimulating choice of our native produce with many refinements, such as named varieties of potatoes, unusual and neglected vegetables like Swiss chard or Jerusalem artichokes and a choice of winter squashes. In place of the standard 'winter lettuce' forced under glass, you'll get good strong lamb's lettuce or land cress. In summer, the sal-adisi mix (see page 19) from a local producer will be far superior to the supermarkets' 'mixed leaf packs', and you will be able to eat those raspberries or strawberries without wondering about the number of chemical treatments they have received.

There will be no unnecessary packaging, you'll have a more direct link with the producers, and you can buy organic vegetables at a fraction of the price in supermarkets and in much better condition.

FRUIT AND VEGETABLE CLASSIFICATIONS

When you see 'Class 1 Produce' on a box or label, you cannot necessarily assume that this is an indicator of quality. The European Union has devised a grading system for all the produce sold in Europe but unfortunately this has very limited guidelines which are geared towards presentation and appearance. Taste, nutritiousness, absence of chemical residues and other consumer concerns are totally ignored.

There are four major classifications for fruit and vegetables in Europe. Top of them all is **Extra Class**. This is reserved for produce of 'superior' quality that has no defects. It is very rarely used and only for specially selected produce, such as perfect peaches and flawless apples. Most of the produce on our shelves these days qualifies for **Class 1**. This grading is given to 'good-quality' produce with no defects. **Class 2** applies to produce that is of 'reasonable' quality but it can be 'deficient' in one or more minor aspects, such as shape, colour or blemishing. Fruit and vegetables of 'marketable' quality which don't meet the other standards are lumped into **Class 3** and usually sold only for food processing or when there is a shortage.

All this sounds sensible until you appreciate that EU classifications are essentially cosmetic ones. To qualify for a Class 1 grade, for example, new carrots must be no smaller than 1 centimetre in diameter and 8 grams in weight. A banana must be at least 14 centimetres long and 27 millimetres in diameter and must not be 'abnormally curved'. In other words, they must be well and truly 'calibrated'.

This obsession with appearance encourages growers to concentrate on produce that is uniform in size and shape and blemish free. As anyone with an allotment, kitchen garden, or experience of orchards knows, fruit and vegetables do not naturally grow in such a standardised way. An apple tree might bear fruit as big as a grapefruit alongside others as small as a rosehip. Carrots can often have a very irregular appearance but still taste really good.

But the EU classifications encourage growers to aim for the visually perfect results that this grading system rewards above other things. This means using more pesticides and artificial inputs and planting generally tasteless 'modern' varieties which have been developed to meet the buying and selling requirements of large multiples and wholesalers – fruit with 'bruise-resistant' skin, and so on. Fewer interesting varieties make their way on to the market and experimentation becomes less likely. A certain type of potato, for example, might produce lots of variable, knobbly-looking tubers but the texture and taste might knock spots off the more readily available varieties. Yet growers nevertheless feel inclined to stick with the same standard product because it is more likely to make the grade. The demands of the consumer who only wants good, safe, wholesome food are simply not taken into account.

FROZEN FRUIT AND VEGETABLES

Frozen fruit and vegetables are always an improvement on tinned ones but how do they compare with fresh? There is a lot of evidence that very fresh fruit and vegetables, frozen at their nutritional peak, retain more vitamins and minerals than so-called 'fresh' produce in shops which might be several days old.

Texture, of course, is a different matter. All fruit and vegetables suffer textural changes when frozen. The most obvious example of this is strawberries, which cannot hold their shape. Even frozen vegetables such as peas and green beans, often recommended as good substitutes for fresh, bear no comparison to their fresh equivalents. As well as feeling different in the mouth they produce more water and usually adversely affect a dish.

Frozen summer fruits have their uses, in purées, sauces and so on where the taste matters, not the texture. Two frozen vegetables – spinach and corn – are reasonably good stand-ins for fresh. Apart from these, frozen fruit and vegetables promise much and deliver little, even at difficult times of the year when fresh produce is at its lowest ebb.

How to choose fruit

This is largely a question of finding fruit that is ripe, the best guarantee you can have that it will taste good. Ripe fruit is at its nutritional peak, with its acids and sugars in good equilibrium. Because it gives off volatile aromas (scent), you should be able to judge whether a fruit is ripe by smelling it.

Certain basic criteria come before scent. The fruit should look appetising but any irregularity in size or shape – providing it isn't too extreme – is fine. Avoid any fruit that is badly squashed, has rotten bits or a wrinkled skin.

A TROUBLESHOOTING GUIDE

Missing central stalks (apples, pears): A sign of weakness. The fruit is more likely to be rotten inside.
Matt khaki-coloured patches or 'russeting' like russet apples (plums, pears, non-russet apples): Considered as a fault by conventional growers, but this superficial blemish has no effect on taste or texture.
Sticky blobs of transparent, gluey matter (plums): The skin has been pierced by a very small insect and the sap has come out and formed around the point. Growers see it as a minor fault but

it can be simply knocked off and won't affect eating quality, unless the damage is extensive.

Bruising (nectarines, apricots, apples, pears): The fruit has been damaged and the flavour will be affected. The bad bits can be cut out and the rest salvaged but there is a risk that the whole fruit is infected by harmful bacteria.

Splitting (cherries, melons): A sign of overripeness. The fruit may still taste okay once the split has been removed, but since it has been weakened it is more likely to become rotten and be colonised by bacteria, which could be harmful.

Furry skins (peaches): Not a fault. Some varieties, mainly traditional ones, just have thicker, furrier skins!

Whiteish bloom (plums, blueberries): Normal on certain varieties.

Whiteish powder on leaves or fruits, unusual odour (strawberries, raspberries): Dangerous; possibly residues of chemicals sprayed too close to harvest. Phone up your local Environmental Health or Trading Standards Office and ask them to test the fruit for you. Alert whoever sold it to you.

JUDGING RIPENESS

There is nothing more irritating than fruit that fails to ripen as it should. Although selecting even staple fruits like pears can sometimes be difficult, the fruits that usually disappoint are summer varieties such as peaches and melons. To add insult to injury, because these are generally imported they are invariably expensive. So not only does that nectarine or melon turn out to be a woolly or turnipy duffer which is entirely useless (unless, of course, you want to play rounders with it) but it also represents a significant amount of money down the drain. Not the sort of experience that's likely to encourage the nationwide increase in fruit consumption that health experts insist is so necessary!

Aroma is the best guide to ripeness for most fruit, and generally to flavour. So for fruits that are notoriously difficult to judge –

melons, peaches, nectarines, pineapples, strawberries – use your nose. All these fruits should smell fresh, remind you of the flavours you would associate with them (even if you were blindfolded) and make you want to eat them. Pick them up (ignore any dirty looks from shop assistants) and sniff them. If they smell of nothing, don't buy them. They are either immature, underripe, or have been so over-refrigerated to stop them rotting that they will never have any flavour or scent. Fruits with perfumes that make you think of boiled sweets such as pineapple chunks or fruit pastilles are overripe and may be almost fermenting. It is touch and go whether these will taste good or be just a bit too 'high'.

There are other tests for specific fruit. In the case of **melons**, press the base to see if it gives and wiggle the stalk around gently; if it separates a little, the melon is likely to be good. For **pineapple**, look for a nice even, yellow-to-slightly-green exterior without any trace of grey. For **peaches**, squeeze the stalk end gently; it should give slightly.

Even harder fruits, such as **apples and pears**, should have a lighter but nevertheless distinct aroma of fruit. Fruit such as **mangoes, kiwis and papayas** do not smell, but should be firm and even to the touch, without any black spots or rot but with a slight 'give' under the skin. Unripe kiwis will be hard inside, difficult to spoon out and probably too acid – leave them until they slacken off a bit. Mangoes and papayas are often ripe inside when they still seem hard outside – don't leave them too long.

Water melons should sound hollow when tapped. **Bananas** should be yellow rather than green, but not too smelly. The only way to judge if fruit such as **grapes, blueberries, raspberries and gooseberries** are ripe is to taste them.

Size matters with stone fruits such as peaches, nectarines, apricots, cherries, plums and greengages. Larger fruits tend to be riper, since they have spent longer on the tree and soaked up more sun – that makes them sweeter. There is an exception – all those fat, black plums that are imported from the USA and countries like Chile have been bred to yield large, firm fruits which stand up to long transport. Evidence indeed that big is not always best!

Green and 'backward' fruit

Although the UK – and England in particular – once had extensive orchards producing fruit such as apples, plums, cherries and pears, we are no longer a great fruit-producing nation. This means that few of us have the opportunity, as consumers in other parts of the world do, to buy fruit at its peak of ripeness.

Since we rely on imports for much of our fruit, and are often fairly clueless about judging its quality, the wholesale fruit trade, aided and abetted by our large food retailers, has developed a form of retailing that eliminates risk. It is customary in Britain to sell certain fruits in a state known as green and 'backward'. In other words, the fruit is not ripe.

Fruit retailed in this way has great appeal for both the grower and the retailer. It is usually mechanically harvested when it is still hard, which is much cheaper than the hand picking that would be necessary if the fruit was approaching true ripeness. Since, unlike trained human pickers, machines are not selective, whole fields or orchards can be 'strip-picked' at the same time. This means, inevitably, that ripe and underripe fruit are harvested together. All fruit, whether it is grown on the same patch of soil or the same tree, will ripen at a different rate according to how much sunlight it gets.

Wholesalers like fruit that has been harvested green and backward – first, because it is cheap and secondly because it is easy to handle, standing up to routine packing and haulage without showing obvious signs of trauma. Underripe fruit offers retailers a much better shelf life, so there are less likely to be 'returns' – fruit sent back after being rejected.

And what does the consumer get? If you are lucky, fruit that may ripen eventually. But in the case of fruit that has been picked so immature that the basic ripening process has been halted, or has been badly stored, you end up with specimens that are both underripe and rotten at the same time – a double insult. Our large food suppliers justify selling fruit in this unripe state on the basis that 'the housewife' (always a term used when they want to hood-wink and patronise us) prefers to shop only once a week, and therefore fruit must be underripe so that 'she' can buy it on Thursday and keep it until the following Wednesday. 'And any-way,' so the argument goes, 'it may be underripe but it is mature, and so it will ripen up in your fruit bowl.'

As experience will probably tell you, this is absolute nonsense. While, in theory, it is possible for fruit to be harvested when it is *mature* but not entirely ripe, and then subsequently ripen over a period of days, this requires quite strict controls. Fruit at this stage needs an atmosphere that is fairly warm but also damp and humid. Most modern homes are far too hot and dry for fruit to ripen, especially in the kitchen where it is most likely to be stored.

'Ripe and ready' labels

In response to complaints about the uselessness of green and back-ward fruit, there has been a spate of new labels in supermarkets – 'ripe and ready' or 'ready to eat', which appears to offer consumers a guarantee that the fruit is in prime condition for eating and that no further ripening at home is required.

The idea is that fruit is allowed to mature on the tree or in the field. The same tree or patch might be picked over selectively up to eight times by skilled pickers, whose job it is to make sure that each batch of fruit is at the same stage of maturity. These fruits are then transported at very carefully regulated temperatures and sold quickly, since they have a much shorter shelf life. Compared to green and backward fruit, this is a high-risk operation. In theory, the fruit should taste very much more like the luscious fruit we associate with sunny, Continental markets.

Fruit sold under these labels costs significantly more than ordinary produce. Usually they are very large, extremely good-looking specimens, which are specially packaged to prevent damage while they are in this more vulnerable, truly ripe condition.

This type of labelling was pioneered by Marks and Spencer, who, since it caters for the last-minute rather than the once-a-week shopper, recognised that consumers wanted to buy fruit to eat the same day. While they have managed to offer fruit that generally fits the bill – albeit at a price – the same cannot be said for the supermarket chains that have unashamedly copied these labels. Because they are geared up to once-a-week shopping, they find ripe-and-ready fruit difficult to handle, and generally their offerings are an expensive disappointment, displaying a range of faults from mushiness through to a total absence of flavour. If you buy produce like this, take it back to the store, if you have the energy, or write a letter of complaint. Failing that, avoid these labels entirely – you can probably buy better at a fraction of the cost in your local greengrocer's.

FRUIT WITH LEAVES ON

It is becoming more common to see fruit – usually lemons, clementines and other citrus fruit – with the leaves still attached. This is the grower's way of indicating that it has been freshly harvested – a guarantee of 'new-season' fruit. If it wasn't fresh, the leaves would have gone dry and fallen off. Since citrus fruit is often stored for months at a time, and sold without leaves, leaves attached are a reliable indicator of freshness.

How to choose vegetables, salad leaves and herbs

The key issue when selecting vegetables, salad leaves and herbs is **freshness**. This is usually quite easy to judge. Green vegetables and leaves should have a vibrant colour. All vegetables should look full of vitality and smell good. Mould, rot and sliminess of any kind is always unacceptable. Flabbiness, a tendency to bend and feel rubbery (cauliflower or cucumber, for example), wrinkling and wilting are out.

As a general rule, **shape** is secondary. Oddly shaped, twisted, irregularly sized vegetables can all be fine, but this is a question of degree. A little abnormality is acceptable but a very abnormally shaped carrot, for example, has grown badly and will not have absorbed its intake of nutrients in a balanced way.

When it comes to **size**, small is not always beautiful. Baby vegetables came into fashion a few years back and still account for a large amount of shelf space in supermarkets. But with the notable exception of cherry tomatoes, which do generally taste sweeter and have a better texture than larger tomatoes, small vegetables taste of very little – and cost a lot.

Some baby vegetables offer a welcome tenderness, especially when winter vegetables are past their best. But baby carrots, for example, cannot match the strong, developed flavour of dark-orange winter carrots. Fine varieties of green beans may look even and regular and lend themselves to presentation in cute little parcels bound with chives, but they do not have the depth of flavour found in larger, more mature beans. Extra-thin baby asparagus may sound great, but larger, fatter stems have a much more three-dimensional taste.

Although we associate baby vegetables with spring and fresh new crops, the baby vegetable industry is a year-round enterprise, so many of the crops have to be grown fairly artificially in glasshouse conditions. As a result, though they look very pretty, the eating experience usually disappoints.

A TROUBLESHOOTING GUIDE

Holes in leaves (lettuce, cabbage, broccoli): A sign of pest activity. You may have to wash off some little blighters but the holes won't harm you.

Sprouting (onions, garlic, lettuce, brassicas): Avoid. Last-ditch attempt of the plant to reproduce, which changes chemical composition and therefore flavour.

Potato sprouting: As above, but if the potato is still firm the sprouts can be knocked off and the potato may still taste good. It can be a positive sign that the potato has not been treated with chemical sprout-inhibitor. (See page 29.)

Dirt (potatoes, carrots, lettuce): This simply means the vegetables have not been washed. As long as the dirt is sweet and fresh smelling, it's fine. If it is slimy or sulphurous, avoid.

Long cut marks (potatoes): A sign of careless mechanical harvesting. Cuts weaken and expose the potato to rot. A matter of degree – the odd mark is acceptable, more than that is not.

Rubberiness (potatoes, carrots, parsnips, cauliflowers): A sign that the vegetables are too old or have been badly stored. Avoid.

Green patches (potatoes, carrots). Poisonous natural toxins. Avoid.

Whiteish bloom (cabbages and other brassicas): Certain varieties have a natural bloom. You can tell when it is natural because it does not rub off with your finger. A powdery residue from spraying would rub off at least a little.

Whiteish powder on leaves and/or unusual odour (lettuce, leafy vegetables): Dangerous; possibly residues of chemicals sprayed too close to harvest. Phone up your local Environmental Health or Trading Standards Office and ask them to test it. Alert whoever you bought it from.

HERBS AND SALAD LEAVES – FINDING THE RIGHT SUPPLY

Over recent years, supermarkets have taken to selling a wide range of herbs and salad leaves on a year-round basis. However, like fruit and vegetables, herbs and salad leaves have their natural seasons too. That's summer for conventional salad leaves – Little Gem, Cos, oak-leaf lettuce and curly endive – and for green leafy herbs such as mint, coriander and basil. Out of the summer and early-autumn period, most of these will be grown in glasshouses.

There are some winter salads, such as lamb's lettuce, dandelions and certain cresses, and hardier herbs like rosemary, thyme, bay and sage can sometimes keep going all year round in ideal circumstances.

Obviously the best way to keep yourself in herbs or salad leaves is to **grow them** in the garden or in a pot on the windowsill. Don't try to do this with the pot herbs (see below) that you can now buy in supermarket produce departments. This is a waste of time. Buy nice, strong, vigorous ones from a market gardener and pot them up in proper earth.

Failing this, buy direct from **farm-gate or organic vegetable box schemes**, which will keep you supplied with seasonal herbs and salad leaves. Many grow what is known as 'misticanza' or 'saladisi' – a mixture of cut-and-come-again salad leaves which is best in the summer but can nevertheless offer something green and leafy throughout most of the year. Some **ethnic stores** are good sources of generous bunches of imported herbs such as mint and coriander, sold loose.

Herbs sold in **pre-packs** are an exceedingly expensive way to buy. In summer, when the less hardy herbs like basil are in profusion, these packs offer small quantities at a high mark-up. In winter, the same pre-packs are stuffed with either expensive airfreighted herbs (often Israeli) or glasshouse herbs (see page 30). Neither tends to be particularly pungent or aromatic.

Many cut herbs are 'gas-flushed' in their packs with nitrogen and carbon dioxide gas. This is known as 'controlled' or 'modified' atmosphere packaging, and has the effect of slowing down the deterioration of the leaves, thus extending shelf life. There is no evidence that this technology is harmful and it does not need to be declared on the label. However, it lends a counterfeit freshness to herbs that may have been cut some days before and have very little of the flavour you might expect from that herb when it was really fresh and prolific. Salad leaves are routinely packed in the same way inside puffed-up, crinkly bags. They seem to last better than the herbs but the mixture of leaves is often not as interesting or varied as it should be, given the price charged.

Herbs sold in pots are really just a gimmick. They look like better value for money but in fact tend to be worse value than cut herbs – and that is some achievement! Although they may look attractive, they are the product of glasshouses (see page 30), and therefore are bound to disappoint. Seedling herbs are planted in 'substrates', or earth substitutes, and encouraged to grow with artificial heat and light. They stay looking attractive long enough to sell but when you get them home you will find they have none of the vigour of a healthy herb plant potted in earth and will literally fade away. Harvest them once, they'll give you a pallid harvest of amazingly unaromatic growth, then slowly die. A monument to how value-added marketing takes advantage of consumer gullibility.

SELECTING MUSHROOMS

Although they may look different, **button**, **closed cup**, **large flat** and **breakfast mushrooms** are all the same variety, *Agaricus bisporus*, or white mushroom. They have just been picked at different stages of development and therefore show more or less of the gills. **Brown-cap** mushrooms, or **champignons de Paris**, are a slightly different variety which is becoming more available. Many people think it has a better flavour than the more common white mushroom. Certain other types of mushrooms are commonly sold as '**wild**' mushrooms, even though they are now widely cultivated just like white ones. These include **shiitake** and **oyster** mushrooms. The latter may be grey, white, yellow, pink or violet, but they are still just oyster mushrooms.

Cultivated 'wild' mushrooms are not noted for their flavour. Shiitake have a slightly garlicky taste, while oyster mushrooms taste of very little. For true wild mushroom flavour, you need to find the best varieties – **chanterelle** (*Cantharius cibarius*), **cep** (*Boletus edulis*) and **morel** (*Morchella esculenta* and *vulgaris*). These are never cultivated and are only available fresh from specialist food shops during their season, or dried out of season.

Out in the wild, mushrooms grow naturally in dark, shady conditions on vegetative material such as tree bark and roots. The cultivated mushrooms you see in the shops are grown in circumstances that mimic this environment. The basic material in most commercial mushroom growing is a compost made up from straw and pig and horse manure. A minority of growers also use a small proportion of processed waste from poultry (faeces, feathers, dead birds and old straw) known as DPM – dried poultry manure. Mushroom spores are inoculated into a grain, usually rye, and this is distributed into the prepared pasteurised compost in warm, damp, dark growing houses. A 'mycelium' develops and the mushrooms appear in flushes over a number of weeks.

Though there is nothing sinister about the idea of growing fungi in this way, two issues need to be borne in mind. The first is the type of compost used. Wastes such as DPM are controversial because it is thought that they might harbour diseases and infectious material from intensive livestock production. The second is that because mushrooms are susceptible to a pest (mushroom fly) and fungal diseases, they are produced with the routine use of chemical insecticides and soil sterilants, many of which are extremely toxic.

One clear alternative for those concerned about pesticides is **organic** mushrooms, which are now widely available at a reasonable price. In organic mushroom production, DPM is banned and all waste must come from approved sources. The chemicals approved for use in conventional mushroom production are not permitted and only insecticides of natural origin, such as pyrethrins, are used. The emphasis is on biological, physical and barrier methods of pest control, plus a general emphasis on preventative hygiene using techniques such as steam sterilisation.

SELECTING TOMATOES

A good tomato should be a deep, intense red colour and very firm to the touch. It should smell seductively of tomato and make you want to eat it. In the mouth, there should be a perfect balance of two elements – sugar and acid. The first comes from the tomato's exposure to sun, the second from good feeding and therefore the right intake of nutrients. The flavour should explode in your mouth. Firmness is important. Soft or mushy tomatoes are either gorged with water or overripe. In practice, the tomatoes most likely to fit the bill in Britain on a year-round basis are **smaller varieties** – often cherry. This is because although it is possible to grow larger tomatoes with a good flavour it is much easier to produce small ones that taste good. Very large tomatoes may look like the ones sold in Mediterranean markets but they are nearly always picked too soon, in order to sell them in good condition, and so the flavour doesn't live up to the promise.

With tomatoes of all sizes, the most important factor is their ripeness when picked. Most tomatoes we buy in Britain (mainly Dutch and, to a lesser extent, home produced) are picked green and unripe, then artificially ripened in special chambers with ethylene gas – the gas that ripe fruit gives off naturally. These tomatoes tend to have rather pallid pink skin and rosy flesh. The flavour is similar to a slightly sweet water bomb. They aren't worth eating.

Increasingly, more tomatoes are being sold on the vine to show that they have not been artificially ripened. These remain in good condition for longer, are nice and red and maintain more flavour. So vine-ripened tomatoes can be well worth the extra price.

More elongated varieties – **plum tomatoes** – often look better than the standard glasshouse offerings. They tend to have a higher dry-matter content than round tomatoes and so are less watery. This is why they are popular for canning – the purpose for which they were developed. They don't always have a good flavour though, and rarely compare with a well-grown, properly ripened round variety.

Tomatoes that have been grown outdoors can have a very good flavour because they have to struggle a bit harder to grow and take longer to reach maturity.

The source of a tomato is often a useful indicator of how good it will taste. As a general rule, the further south and closer to the sun you go, the better the tomato. So southern Italian (especially Sicilian), Canary Islands and Moroccan tomatoes are good bets. French tomatoes can be great at the peak of the summer. Though there are still some very decent Jersey and Scottish tomatoes, they lack the sweetness of tomatoes from hot, sunny countries.

More varieties of tomatoes are coming on to the market, the most successful of which are **Gardener's Delight, Cherry Delight** and **Melrow**. However, variety may be something of a diversion, since the growing method and, most importantly, the amount of sun, seem to be the most significant factors in producing tomatoes with flavour. So, buy red, buy firm, favour small, favour Southern.

WHAT HAPPENED TO THE SEASONS?

Fruit and vegetables always taste best in season, when they are sold very soon after harvesting. If, like many shoppers, your grasp on seasons has always been quite vague, by now you are probably well and truly confused. Common sense tells us that apples are picked in the autumn and strawberries in the summer but the old adage about there being a season for everything no longer seems to apply, because just about everything is on offer all year round.

This is because the fruit and vegetable buyers for our large importers and supermarket chains spend their days chasing the sun around the world, in search of climates that can produce fruit and vegetables at times when they would be otherwise unobtainable or taste awful. Raspberries at Christmas, apples in June, and sugar-snap peas in March are just three examples of the global sourcing that allows us to choose from a wider range of fruit and vegetables than ever before.

Global sourcing is undoubtedly here to stay, but that does not mean that consumers should give up looking for seasonal foods. The problem is trying to figure out the season, since many fruit and vegetables are stored (this is discussed in more detail on page 26). And since a harvesting date is not demanded by law, we have no way of knowing exactly when produce has been harvested. Odd clues (such as 'new' on potatoes) tell us that certain produce is fresher than others, but advances in storage techniques make it possible for fruit and vegetables to look fresh when they are in fact several months old.

You can use a rudimentary grasp of British seasons and world geography to figure out what might be seasonal in other parts of the world. Since Britain is in the northern hemisphere, our seasons are a mirror image of the southern hemisphere. Our apples, for example, would normally crop in our autumn (October–December), while New Zealand apples would normally crop in their autumn, which means May, June and July. Should you be buying apples in summer, therefore, buy ones from the southern hemisphere rather than British or French. Likewise, if it is coming up to Christmas, stick with a northern hemisphere apple which, though stored, will be much fresher than, say, a Chilean apple, which has probably been stored for anything up to eight months.

Another good example of this principle is oranges. The European and North African season (e.g. Spain, Morocco) is November to May, while the southern hemisphere season (e.g. South Africa, Argentina) is June to October. So if you were looking for oranges in October, the southern hemisphere ones would be the freshest. Developments in glasshouse horticulture (see page 30) and research into early and late varieties are extending European seasons all the time. French strawberries from Carpentras start coming on to the market in February. Spanish nectarines and peaches, first early, then mid and finally late varieties, may be available as early as April and continue until October.

This season-extension is particularly appealing in early spring, when local produce can be at its lowest ebb. But patience does pay out in the end. Few of these extended-season fruit and vegetables are flavoursome and they are bound to be expensive. None can compete with produce grown at the traditional peak of that particular growing season. Buy them if you are desperate but remember that as little as a fortnight later, they will taste sweeter and cost less.

THE ARRIVAL OF EXOTICS

Peruvian mangoes, Thai asparagus, Nigerian mangetout, Madagascan lychees and Colombian pitahayas. These are just a few of the exotic fruit and vegetables that now find their way on to supermarket shelves. Most of them are flown in by the principle of piggy-backing – that is, on regular airline flights rather than cargo-only planes. The idea is that this cuts costs and makes air-freighting economically viable.

When you are shopping, it is important to make a distinction between exotics that come by air and those that come by sea. Air-freight is reserved for fruits (such as raspberries) and vegetables (such as green beans and peas) that do not ripen once they have been picked or store well. This is a high-risk market and there-fore the produce is likely to be fresh, if frighteningly expensive. Items such as mangoes, papayas and pineapples which can be shipped may also be air-freighted if they have been picked ripe. They will cost anything up to four times the usual price, but will almost certainly taste much better.

Fruit brought by sea (pineapples, bananas, mangoes, grapes and so on) are usually picked underripe so they can survive longer in transit, and they tend to have extra fungicides applied for the same reason (see page 29). When they arrive at their destination they are moved into ripening chambers, where ethylene gas is used to simulate a gigantic fruit bowl effect and ripen them. Results vary from quite good to dreadful, but they cost much less than their air-freighted equivalents.

Storage – how fresh is 'fresh'?

Some fruit and vegetables, such as strawberries and asparagus, have such a short shelf life that it is impossible to store them. Others, particularly apples, cabbage, citrus fruit, onions, pears and pota-toes, can be stored for months. Storing is something that has been going on for centuries. Traditional ways to store include wrap-ping apples up in paper, stacking them gently on top of each other, then leaving them in a dark attic or barn. Potatoes and carrots were dug up and put into thick sacks which allowed no light, while onions were dried and hung up on the rafters of airy barns. Since farms and houses were cold, produce stored in this way could keep from autumn harvest through to the spring. Quite a lot of emphasis was put on choosing varieties – a selection of early, maincrop and late – so that the harvest could be staggered. Certain early varieties of potatoes keep well until Christmas and deteriorate rapidly thereafter. Obvious signs include sprouting but less evident changes affect the texture, and even taste. Old potatoes can taste almost sweet because the starch has begun to convert to sugar. Garlic can literally turn to dust.

A low temperature, and darkness, can help conserve many fruit and vegetables. Citrus fruit will keep for months if stored in cardboard boxes and refrigerated. Developments in modern agriculture and conservation technology mean that it is increasingly feasible to enhance the shelf life of certain fruit and vegetables. With the aid of chemical inputs, modern varieties can produce visually perfect fruit and vegetables which will stay looking that way long after they have been separated from their life source.

COSMETIC WAXES

Some fruit and vegetables, including apples, pears, cucumbers and all citrus fruits, are routinely waxed to prevent wrinkling, thus improving their appearance and extending their shelf life. Even if a fruit or vegetable has not had any post-harvest chemical treatment, it can still be waxed. The waxes are a glazing agent called shellac (the secretions of a tropical insect) and carnauba wax, which is derived from a type of palm tree. Both are thought to be harmless. Any wax is, of course, a purely cosmetic treatment to help produce look fresher and finer longer. A benefit to the wholesaler perhaps, but positively misleading for the consumer.

CONTROLLED-ATMOSPHERE STORAGE AND GAS RIPENING

Most apples are routinely kept in large, computer-controlled chambers in what is called 'controlled-atmosphere storage'. Ordinary air is made up of 80 per cent nitrogen, 20 per cent oxygen and 0.3 per cent carbon dioxide. If apples were left out in this, their skins would shrink, making them look old, and they would eventually rot. But by reducing the oxygen element to 3 per cent and increasing the nitrogen and carbon dioxide to 95 per cent and 2 per cent respectively, it is possible to slow down the respiration rate of the apples. This technology has the effect of significantly extending the shelf life of foods, by anything from two to five times, depending on the product. And because controlled-atmosphere storage is regarded as just a variation on the natural composition of air, it does not have to be mentioned on the label. Bananas, too, are increasingly being kept in this way. They are picked green, stored in a controlled atmosphere, then ethylene-gassed to ripen them when they are needed. Some potatoes get the same treatment.

The advantages of this system for growers and wholesalers is obvious. A large harvest can be purchased all at once, stored and then put out on the shelves as required. From the consumer's point of view, though, the system amounts to deception, since it bestows a counterfeit freshness. Trusting and naive souls that we are, we tend to think that everything we buy is fresh, though some of us do wonder how strange countries are managing to produce certain crops at odd times of the year!

Although stored produce might look good, it has often subtly changed for the worse. The most everyday examples of this are apples that have become floury and grainy in texture, potatoes that seem watery and fall apart when cooked, and bananas that have no flavour.

Storage technology also has a generally pernicious effect on our food supply. Large supplies of standard, boring varieties are a safe bet for wholesalers and retailers. This makes them less interested in buying fleeting supplies of more interesting produce. After all, a short-term source might cause administrative problems and confuse the computer! Farmers soon get the message that variety and experimentation are risky, and this promotes conservatism amongst them. Growing an apple that stores well becomes a more important commercial consideration than producing one that tastes good.

CONSERVATION WITH POST-HARVEST CHEMICALS

However unseductive controlled-atmosphere storage might seem, it pales in comparison with the standard chemical approaches to extending shelf life. Take potatoes. Even stored in the cold and dark, these would eventually sprout – the potato's way of indicating that it is beginning to deteriorate. The standard method of dealing with this is to treat them with Tecnazene, a toxic fungicide that inhibits sprouting. Because this is applied at what is deemed to be a 'safe' interval before sale, it does not need to be declared on the label. In practice, many European supermarkets nevertheless post up notices indicating which potatoes have been treated with a sprout suppressant. In Britain, this is unheard of.

Citrus fruit, bananas, apples, pears, cherries and grapes are routinely treated with chemical preservatives post-harvest to delay spoilage during transport and storing. These are substantially different from chemicals used in the course of growing a crop. In theory, these will have disappeared, while post-harvest chemicals are very definitely sitting there on the skin.

The most common of these is Thiabendazole, which is banned in the USA. Others, such as Diphenyl, Orthophenylphenol and Sodium orthophenylphenate are highly suspect as human carcinogens or mutagens. Although these preservatives have 'E' numbers (E230–233) which would have to be included on the ingredients listing in other food products, fruit and vegetables are mysteriously exempt from such labelling requirements. Nevertheless, in many European countries and in the USA these treatments are indicated at the point of sale. In the UK, however, these additives are not declared either on the label or by way of a sign above loose produce, and so remain invisible to the consumer.

The solution is to buy organic fruits or those that say 'without post-harvest treatment' on the label. These are essential if you want to use the citrus rind in cooking. If you have to buy treated citrus fruit, don't use the rind. After peeling clementines, oranges, etc., or bananas, wash your hands in warm soapy water.

CAN YOU WASH OFF A RESIDUE?

If fruit and vegetables have been grown with chemicals or given post-harvest treatments, the theory is that these should have disappeared by the time you eat them. But spot checks find residues in excess of government limits with depressing regularity. The government says that carrots, for instance, need to be topped generously and then peeled to limit exposure to residues. Even then, only four-fifths of residues from the most toxic organophosphorous chemicals will be removed. This does not include ones that are systemic – contained within the flesh of the fruit or vegetable – or the numerous non-organophosphate chemical treatments that are commonly used. Some shops now sell wax-removing soap products that claim to wash off and eliminate post-harvest treatments, but it is not clear how effective they are. Some chemicals are reduced or destroyed by cooking.

For anyone who likes to eat fruit and vegetables raw, with their nutritious skins intact, the most positive approach is to eat organic.

Glasshouse growing

Most consumers think of vegetables growing in fields. These days, though, many of the vegetables we eat – such as cucumber, peppers, lettuce, aubergine, radishes, tomatoes, and strawberries – are grown in glasshouses. Even fruits such as melons are mainly grown commercially under glass or plastic.

The basic principle is familiar to any gardener. The glass traps the heat of the sun and creates a warmer atmosphere. This protects the plants and allows the gardener to grow crops that might otherwise be impossible to raise outdoors at that time of year. It also means the gardener can extend the natural seasons for plants, 'bringing on' familiar crops so that they can be harvested earlier, or planting later than usual in order to have an extended harvest.

Modern horticulture has developed the basic greenhouse principle almost out of all recognition. The pioneers in this field are the Dutch but there is also extensive glasshouse production in other Northern European countries such as Belgium and, to a lesser extent, the UK.

For the grower, the attraction of this type of horticulture is obvious. Glasshouses, in theory anyway, allow growers to overcome the limitations imposed on them by their location and climate. You wouldn't normally be able to grow a red pepper in Holland in March, for example. The glasshouse opens up the possibility of almost year-round production of staple fruit and vegetables and this strengthens the grower's market position.

For the consumer, however, the benefits are not so straightforward. Glasshouse vegetables are not grown in the traditional sense of the word but are technically induced. The difference between this kind of crop and one grown out of doors in more natural circumstances is immense. Glasshouse horticulture varies from grower to grower but a common approach is as follows. A variety of plant is chosen which is 'adapted' to indoor growing, usually a modern hybrid variety which is known to produce a large yield and be visually attractive. That means shiny and regular in size. The seedlings are then planted in soil substitutes, known as 'substrates'. The most common of these are rockwool, which looks rather like the materials used for packaging and stuffing cushions, and coir, which is otherwise used for tough floor matting. These inert and sterile substances are used to support the roots of the plant while liquid nutrients are pumped into it, a system sometimes known as 'hydroponics'. The nutrients are meant to feed the plant the liquid equivalent of what they would normally take up from the soil – nitrogen, potassium, minerals and so on. In some systems, the plants are rooted in hanging bags containing peat or substrates, irrigated and fed through a hose pipe.

Crops grown by these techniques are so artificial that a cocktail of chemicals must also be fed to them to achieve the intended results: chemical fertilisers to accelerate plant growth, chemical growth regulators, and fungicides to protect these extremely sensitive crops from disease.

Since the crops are literally being tricked into growing, and at a vastly accelerated pace, a constant temperature is required. Some also need special lighting. So greenhouses have to be air-conditioned and, in some cases, even lit up to simulate sunlight. All this is of great concern to environmentalists because it is an astonishingly energy-intensive and wasteful way to grow food.

For those concerned with taste and flavour, this sort of technique produces vegetables that may look good but are thoroughly artificial. Fruit and vegetables grown in natural circumstances develop flavour because they have been 'stressed' as part of the natural struggle to grow. Glasshouse vegetables have been deprived of that. And however much advocates of glasshouse horticulture try to persuade us otherwise, food that has been artificially induced indoors can never compare with food that has been grown in rich, healthy soil and sunlight, in its natural season.

There are some less extreme variations on glasshouse growing. Some growers still grow in soil but this may be a mixed blessing, since chemical inputs used both to grow the crop and to sterilise the soil afterwards linger on and slowly find their way into our water supply and the food chain. Unacceptable residues of chemicals have been found in spot checks on winter lettuces grown in soil under glass. Other growers buy in soil to grow their crops. Often peat is used and this can be a problem for the environment too, since we may well be using up this precious resource more quickly than the land can make it.

In sunnier countries, heating and air-conditioning may not be needed, depending on the time of year. Within a glasshouse, the feeding regime can be altered to promote slower growth and chemical inputs can be slightly reduced. Thus tomatoes grown in a glasshouse in the sunny Canary Islands will probably taste sweeter than those from Holland. Some producers are trying to introduce more biological controls (see page 282) to cut down the use of chemical inputs.

One quite acceptable variant on the old greenhouse principle is the poly-tunnel. Widely used, even in organic production, it is just what is sounds – a simple polythene protection for plants which is no more sinister than the allotment gardener's cloche! If you buy your vegetables in the local greengrocer's, you might be able to identify glasshouse produce by the box, which may be marked 'glasshouse growers' or a similar variation. In supermarkets there is no way of telling, unless the label states explicitly otherwise – for example 'French Outdoor Tomatoes'.

If you want to avoid glasshouse produce, buy seasonally. Classic Mediterranean produce such as peppers or aubergines imported from Northern Europe in December will inevitably be from a glasshouse. The same applies to British lettuces in March, 'early' British strawberries in May and so on. You will have to use your common sense and grasp of the seasons because you won't find that information on the label.

Vanishing variety and why it matters

That old cliché about variety being the spice of life has a particular relevance when it comes to fruit and vegetables. These days, the choice available in shops might lead you to believe that we have a better range than ever before. Our grandmothers never had kiwis or mangoes, sweet potatoes or mangetout. And they ate a diet that was undeniably more restricted than ours.

However, the increasing availability of these 'new' fruits and vegetables should not blind us to the fact that in a slow, steady, almost invisible way, we are losing the rich heritage of plant diversity that farmers have been building up since history began. Environmentalists call it 'genetic erosion'. To you or me, it means that the fruit and vegetables we eat are becoming more and more uniform. How does this show itself? The most obvious examples are **disappearing species** such as medlars and quinces. Once commonplace in Britain, these are now almost unobtainable unless you collect them in the wild. The rich, tart damson plum is yet another fruit that may well be doomed to the same fate. Though still in production in a few areas, it is becoming harder and harder to find.

The next measure is the dwindling number of **varieties** available within each species. For instance, the UK Apple Register records more than 6,000 varieties but just nine of these account for the bulk of commercial production. It's the same story everywhere. In France, for example, almost three-quarters of apple production are given over to one variety – the misleadingly named Golden Delicious – which just has to be the most boring apple imaginable. In India, farmers used to plant up to 30,000 different varieties of rice but the Indian Agricultural Research Unit estimates that within the next 10 to 15 years just ten varieties will cover 75 per cent of the country's rice-producing area.

Also worrying is the **genetic similarity** of new hybrid varieties of fruit and vegetables coming on to the market. Although they may sound exciting and varied, most of them have one common parent in their pedigree which makes them terribly similar genetically and much of a muchness to eat.

WHY WE NEED BIODIVERSITY

It is obviously in the consumer's interest to see that true variety, or biodiversity, of fruit and vegetables is safeguarded. The first reason is food security. When crops are too similar genetically they are vulnerable to disease. The notorious Irish potato famine of the 1840s is the classic example of this. Because growers had been cultivating potatoes descended from only two key varieties, the entire crop was wiped out by disease.

The second reason is preserving our plant heritage. Once our rich genetic inheritance of plant food is gone it cannot be recreated, and one day we may need it badly. Without this heritage, we surrender the diversity of our food chain to a brave new world, where the same standard crops dominate global agriculture.

Thirdly, biodiversity guarantees taste and flavour. Consumers are sick and tired of cosmetic fruit and vegetables which look the same and share the same, generally bland flavours and standard texture. The reason so many modern varieties often disappoint is that they have been designed for buying and selling. Their role is to make big profits for the large corporations who breed them and to be convenient for the wholesalers and retailers who handle them, not to stimulate the palate of the consumer. These new, standard varieties have emerged because the nature of plant breeding has changed radically. Traditionally, plant breeding consisted of growers and specialist seed companies saving their best seed from one harvest to another, maintaining a supply of tried-and-trusted crops that were well adapted to their local growing circumstances. Modern plant breeding, on the other hand, is controlled by a handful of large pharmaceutical companies who want to see their particular varieties dominate the world market. Increasingly, more and more emphasis is being put on 'super-seeds'. These new strains of crops guarantee large yields and are also dependent on the chemical products – pesticides, fertilisers and so on – of the companies that bred them. These same companies are in the business of picking up varieties from areas of genetic diversity in the Third World, perfecting them and claiming they 'own' them, then forbidding their use except for a large payment.

Taste, flavour and true variety are no longer the name of the breeding game. Unless consumers force these considerations up the plant breeders' list of priorities and on to the political agenda they will not be taken into account.

SUPPORTING VARIETY

Support variety and diversity in fruit and vegetables whenever you can. That might mean planting a few unusual seeds in your windowbox or encouraging local growers who might be prepared to experiment with traditional, less commercial varieties by giving them your business. When shopping in greengrocer's and supermarkets, actively favour the less usual varieties and demand an even larger choice.

PAYING ATTENTION TO VARIETIES

Most of us have got into the habit of buying fruit and vegetables just as 'apples', 'carrots' or 'potatoes'. This is about as informed as asking a travel agent for a 'holiday' without specifying the country, beach versus mountains and so on. Inadequate labelling exploits our ignorance. Quite often, produce is sold only by its country of origin, which means that we haven't a clue which variety within that species we are buying. Such information is crucial. You only need to compare the boring Conference pear with the scented and much more appealing William pear to see what a difference variety can make.

Varietal labelling is becoming more common, particularly for fruits where the differences are quite distinct. European regulations demand that all labels for oranges, grapes and plums must state their variety. Varietal labelling should be compulsory on *all* produce, because it helps us build up a picture of which varieties – even allowing for different production methods – tend to offer the best flavour.

As a general rule, the blandest, most boring varieties from a cooking and eating point of view are being churned out by industrial farming methods, where quantity and uniformity are the most important criteria and taste is just an irritating incidental. Flavour-conscious growers put emphasis on varieties.

THE NUTRITIONAL VALUE OF DIFFERENT VARIETIES

Not all varieties of a particular fruit or vegetable have the same nutritional value. One good example is vitamin C in apples.

Variety	Vitamin C per 100 grams
Sturmer	20 mg
Discovery	16 mg
Cox's Orange	9 mg
Russet	8 mg
Worcester	5 mg
Golden Delicious	4 mg
Granny Smith	4 mg
Red dessert	3 mg

This illustrates how the big commercial varieties (Golden, Granny and red) dominating our shelves often offer poorer nutrition than more traditional varieties which are less widely available. The logical conclusion? These modern varieties have been selected because they are high yielding, store well and are easy to retail, not for their intrinsic nutritional value or eating quality.

VARIETIES OF FRUIT WITH THE BEST FLAVOUR

Apples: Cox's Orange (pre-Christmas), Braeburn, Egremont Russet, Elstar, James Grieve (see page 39)
Pears: William, Comice, Abate Fetel, Bosc, Passe Crassana
Strawberries: Cambridge Vigour, Hapill, Elsanta
Raspberries: Glen Prosen, Glen Moy, Malling Jewel
Plums: Victoria, Marjorie Seedling, Mirabelle (golden), Reine Claude (green), damsons

Grapes: Muscat (white), Muscat de Hambourg (black), Flame, Italia

Cherries: Napoleon (yellow/pink), Reverchon, Van, Griotte/Morello (sour variety)

Mangoes: Alfonso, Bangapalli

Apricots: Orange-red varieties, Hunza (dried), larger, redder varieties

Peaches: White varieties are more perfumed and flavoursome than yellow. Redwing (white), Elegant Lady (yellow)

Nectarines: White varieties are more perfumed and flavoursome than yellow. Snow Queen (white), Red Diamond (yellow)

Melons: Orange-red varieties taste best. Charentais, Cantaloupe, Cavaillon-type

Lemons: Amalfi-type, Verna

Oranges: Navel, Maltaise, Valencia (for juice), Moro, Sanguinelli (and other blood varieties)

'Tangerines': Clementines

EATERS OR COOKERS?

The UK is the only country to have sour apple varieties that have been developed especially for cooking. Other countries do not draw a distinction between cooking and eating, or dessert, apples.

British cooking apples include **Howgate Wonder, Grenadier** and **Lord Derby** but the **Bramley** is Britain's favourite. It is habitually recommended for cooking because of three characteristics:

• It contains anything from two to six times more malic acid than other apple varieties. This gives the characteristic sharp, acidic flavour which some people like and also means the apples can be stored for longer.

- It only has about three-quarters of the sugar of eating apples, which makes it sour and slightly tart.
- It has around 20 per cent less dry matter content than most eating apples, which means that it softens or collapses much more easily during cooking.

However, these are advantages only if you want a smooth, sharp-tasting apple purée. Otherwise Bramleys are not marvellous for cooking. They do not hold their shape, they need substantial quantities of sugar to make them palatable and, last but not least, they are unaromatic and relatively flavourless.

Why the success then? Bramleys store well, better than most sweeter, dryer apples, and this makes them a sound commercial choice for growers, who can supply them on a virtual year-round basis. Because of this, Bramleys have benefited from substantial advertising and marketing backing, to the extent that many consumers are convinced that Bramleys are the *only* variety worth cooking. However, many so-called eating varieties are much better for cooking and need no sugar added.

As a general rule, the more acidic an apple is, the more easily it will soften and form a purée. The way in which an apple cooks also depends on when it was picked and how it was stored. Windfall apples and those picked early in their season tend to be sharper than tree-ripe fruit, which contain more sugar. Apples stored in natural circumstances, as opposed to modern modified-atmosphere methods (see page 27) become progressively sweeter as the acidity level drops.

When you need apples that will hold their shape – for a Tarte Tatin, whole baked apples, and so on – boring old **Granny Smith** or **Golden Delicious** are reliable bets. Apples that perform similarly but have more taste and aroma include **Elstar**, **Idared**, **Braeburn**,

Jonagold and **James Grieve**. Sweeter, less acidic varieties with less crunchy flesh, which cook down into good purées, include **Blenheim Orange**, **Ellison's Orange**, **Worcester Pearmain**, **Charles Ross**, **Reinette**, **Cox's Orange**, **Egremont Russet** and **Discovery**. These are all varieties that have intrinsic flavour, whether eaten raw or cooked.

VARIETIES OF VEGETABLES WITH THE BEST FLAVOUR

Potatoes: Pink Fir Apple, Jersey Royals, Kerr's Pink, Desirée, King Edwards (see page 41)
Cabbages: Savoy, January King
Cultivated mushrooms: brown cap, flat or open
Salad leaves: Cos (Romaine), Little Gem and rocket
Peppers: Clovis (thin and tapering)
Squashes: Butternut and Acorn
Avocados: Hass
Broccoli: purple sprouting
Garlic: violet and pink varieties
Onions: shallots and red varieties
Parsley: flat-leaf
Tomatoes: Cherisita (cherry), 'French outdoor', Gardener's Delight, Cherry Delight, very red ones from sunny countries (see page 22)
Peas: Feltham First, Hurst Green Shaft, sugarsnap
Cucumbers: ridge
Courgettes: dark green types
Parsnips: White Gem
Swede: Maigret

AT-A-GLANCE GUIDE TO POTATO VARIETIES

The UK eats more potatoes per head of population than any other European country – and that includes Ireland! A few standard varieties tend to dominate the market but a growing number of unusual or different types are becoming available. This is good news, because the potato is not a jack-of-all-trades. Here is a guide to which potatoes are best for which purpose.

Firm and waxy varieties (good for boiling, salads and frying because they hold their shape): Desirée, Pink Fir Apple, La Ratte, Belle de Fontenay, Charlotte, Carlingford, Nicola, Roseval, Royal Kidney, Jersey Royal, Arran Pilot, Purple Congo, Truffe de Chine, Aura, Linzer Delikatess

Floury and creamy varieties (good for baking and mash because they soften nicely): King Edward, Golden Wonder, Home Guard, Arran Comet, Cara, Pentland Squire, Record, Epicure, Maris Piper, Catriona, Ausonia, Kerr's Pink, Marfona, Romano, Wilja, Santé, Mona Lisa

Dry, firm varieties that crisp well (good for chips and roasting): Golden Wonder, Record, Catriona, Desirée, Pentland Crown, King Edward

Good all-rounders Desirée, Estima, Record, Catriona, Golden Wonder, Charlotte, Pentland Javelin, Ulster Sceptre, King Edward, Wilja, Maris Piper, Santé

Fish and Shellfish

How times have changed. Fish and shellfish used to be taken for granted – good, wholesome, staple food, generally rated lower down the hierarchy than meat. Sometimes we were a bit sniffy about fish, sticking to certain standard white varieties, suspicious of shellfish and scathing about any species we did not know.

Now many species of fish and shellfish have become some of the priciest and most tantalisingly elusive foods around. Because we have plundered the sea in the mistaken belief that its harvests were infinite, over-fishing has badly affected stocks of even our most workaday species. There is talk of whole stretches of water, such as the North Sea, being completely 'fished out' in coming years. Quotas and de-commissioning of boats means that fish is not a commodity on which we can endlessly rely. So prices are up and really good fish is scarce and highly prized. A lovely turbot or brill routinely costs more, weight for weight, than any prime cut of meat. Meanwhile, that relative newcomer – fish farming – is churning out pounds of cheap fish protein as quickly as it can to cash in on the gap.

The story with shellfish is slightly different but every bit as contrary. Just as we have woken up to the fact that our ancestors had a point – some shellfish is actually very good to eat – we see that much of our native stock is being creamed off by an apparently insatiable foreign market, often by-passing our own retail outlets. When we aren't terrified by the price, we wonder about the health risks of eating shellfish from waters that seem increasingly mucked up by all sorts of pollution.

For all these reasons, many consumers have lost any confidence and certainty when it comes to selecting fish and shellfish. A frightening number have given up the ghost entirely – breaded, battered and processed are the only forms in which many people now experience this potentially magnificent food stuff.

Perhaps it is not such a bad thing that fish has been transformed from the poor relation into glittering invitee. When food is cheap it is taken for granted, and we tend to treat it badly. Belatedly, and for all the wrong reasons, fish and shellfish are at last receiving the respect and attention they deserve.

The best strategy for selecting fish these days is one that is both sceptical and openminded at the same time. Save the scepticism for the waves of farmed fish that are flooding our shelves, the relatively tasteless 'exotic' species flown in from the Indian Ocean at great expense, and the reconstituted 'crab' sticks fresh from the freezer which sell as a token gesture towards shellfish. But make the most of the very decent products that modern aquaculture has developed, such as rope-culture mussels and cultivated oysters. React quickly to the fleeting joys of fresh crab, wild salmon and other native species at their peak of perfection. To do that, you have to pay much more than you might expect for certain species of white fish, such as sole, cod and even plaice. Instead of Tuesday-night supper, think treat of the week.

The bonus is that a more adventurous buying policy can lead you to cheaper categories of fish, often mistakenly rated as inferior. When really fresh, species such as mackerel, sardines, whitebait and herring are absolutely wonderful to eat, not to mention extremely healthy. Buying them is worthwhile – it does not mean that you are trading down.

THE STATE OF THE SEA

The North Sea, which is the source of most of our native fish, is nowhere near as clean as it ought to be. As with fisheries the world over, it has become a dumping ground for a number of contaminants. These include sewage waste, toxic substances such as long-persistence pesticides and their breakdown products, poly-chlorinated biphenyls (PCBs), industrial pollution in the form of heavy metals (mercury, lead, cadmium), and dioxins and leaking radiation from nuclear power stations. The long-term effect of this on our marine fish supply is not known, but two separate European tests on sea fish have shown that around 40 per cent of common species such as plaice and sole show signs of pollution-related disease.

With such active pollutants in the marine environment, some consumers may feel that fish is not the attractive proposition it used to be. Fortunately, the sea seems to have a tremendous ability to withstand such onslaughts. There is no evidence to show that deep sea fish is significantly polluted with toxic residues that could harm human health – something of a miracle in the circumstances!

As a general rule, the further out to sea a fish is caught, the cleaner it is likely to be. This is because contaminants there are more likely to be diluted to what are considered to be 'harmless levels'. River estuaries and waters close to heavily populated, industrial coastal areas are the riskiest for fish. This is particularly true of shellfish (see page 70). So most white fish, such as haddock, sole, cod and so on, are very unlikely to be heavily contaminated, although trace residues of toxins may show up in tests.

Ironically, oily fish such as herring and mackerel are statistically more prone than others to pollution from heavy metals, with the biggest concentration in the roes and livers. So precisely the fish that are best for your health because of their high Omega-3 fatty acid content (this is thought to be protective against heart disease, strokes and some inflammatory illnesses) are the most susceptible to contamination. It is a bit drastic to eliminate them permanently from your diet, but pregnant women and people whose immune system has been weakened through age or illness should not eat too much of this type of fish.

Selecting fresh fish

It would be nice if we could take for granted that all the fish on offer on the fishmonger's slab was fresh. The fact is, we can't. Fish deteriorates extremely rapidly, particularly oily fish. A very fresh mackerel is a pleasure, an old mackerel absolutely disgusting. Modern developments in refrigeration and transport mean that fish travels much further these days, and can be kept for much longer without being obviously 'bad' or stinking. But that does not mean that it is positively fresh. Ten-day-old fillets of cod might not taste actively bad but the flavour and texture will be extremely disappointing.

FACTORS THAT AFFECT THE EATING QUALITY OF FISH

Irrespective of whether fish is fresh or frozen, careful handling is the key factor when it comes to eating quality. Much rests on how it has been caught. Fish caught by a rod and line, either at sea or by an angler, is less likely to be harmed than fish that is netted. Certain types of net can bruise and damage fish, particularly if they are kept in the net for too long once caught. Like animals, fish show signs of stress and this can badly affect the eating quality. Careful handling of fish once landed can minimise this.

The timing and manner in which the newly landed fish is refrigerated can also make a huge difference. Careless handling in transport and over- or under-refrigeration can all detract from eating quality.

Fish straight out of the sea and eaten on the day of harvest can be curiously disappointing. Many experts think that the flavour of larger fish (as opposed to shellfish) is best on the second or third day after harvest. The fish should be allowed to go through rigor mortis and a process similar to the hanging that is traditional with red meat. Much research is currently being carried out on pre- and post-harvest handling of fish.

Handling details such as these are part of the hidden history of fish as far as the ordinary consumer is concerned. However, good independent fishmongers generally welcome questions about how they source their fish. They should be able to tell you why they buy fish from one supplier rather than another, whether the fish came from close water or deep-sea boats and so on.

Two factors within the consumer's control also affect the eating quality of fish. First of all, size. As a rule, larger, more mature fish have a better flavour. Young fish have not grown to their full potential and the flavour tends to be undeveloped. The second is whether the fish is sold whole or filleted. Fillets may be convenient but they never have as good a flavour as fish that has been left on the bone. Because whole fish deteriorate faster than fillets, they have to be sold faster. Whole fish are likely to be fresher and are not so commonly frozen.

CHOOSING YOUR FISH MERCHANT

If you are one of the shrinking number of consumers with access to a really first-class fishmonger, then it pays to become a valued regular customer and put your faith in his or her selection. There are certain clues to finding an establishment that fits the bill:

- Good fish shops have a clean, appetising smell of fresh fish but never an unpleasant 'fishiness' or 'whiff'.
- There should always be other customers in the shop, and preferably a queue stretching out of the door at all but the quietest times. Fish needs a rapid turnover.
- The shop should run out of fish and the selection should change from one day to another. A constant supply of all but the most basic fish suggests that some of it has been previously frozen or refrigerated for too long. Fresh fish supplies are fleeting, often erratic, and seasonal.
- Staff should be able to give you chapter and verse on the precise source of the fish, how it travelled to them and how long it has been in the shop. Fudging, or unwillingness to be specific

about anything other than a general guarantee of freshness, is suspicious.
- Staff should have the skills to fillet a fish on the spot or prepare it exactly as you wish.
- There should be a clear demarcation line between cooked and cured fish and fresh wet fish. (Strong odours of smoking or pickling can taint fresh fish sitting in proximity.)
- The shop should smell and look clean and the temperature should be very cold.

AVOIDING BAD FISHMONGERS

Nostalgia for the days when there were three fish merchants to choose from on every high street should not make us automatically select the local fishmonger, or the market fish stall, rather than the supermarket. The best fish shops are a joy to be in, but they are few and far between, as many small, independent fishmongers have deteriorated into outlets for ready-filleted, much handled and traded fish, which is passed down from huge industrial boats, through fish processors to fairly careless wholesalers.

Warning signs that all is not well down your local fish shop are the opposite of the positive criteria listed above. Another big clue is a preponderance of fillets over whole fish, since it is much harder to disguise age and lack of freshness in whole fish (see page 51).

Although fishmongers are subject to checks from the local Environmental Health or Trading Standards Office, these are considerably less regular than the more systematic checks operating in supermarkets. Freezing leftover fish is a terrible temptation for a fish merchant who is struggling for business and cash.

FRAUDULENT AND FANCIFUL LABELS

Ever wondered what 'rock salmon' or 'mock scampi' might be? The chances are it is a fairly ordinary but decent fish that your fishmonger has decided to rename in order to make it more saleable.

Prime candidates include huss, coley (pollack) and gurnard, which produce good, firm fillets of fish, if not a spectacular flavour. Their chief attraction is that they are cheap.

It is not uncommon to see fish renamed in this way and there is no law against it. Take these names with a pinch of salt and don't have too high expectations about what you are getting. Demand to know the species name before you buy it if you don't recognise the fish.

On occasions, opportunistic fishmongers take advantage of consumer ignorance of species. One common example of this is cheaper white fish being passed off as John Dory – a rather special and fine fish which is invariably expensive. This is not a 'mistake' that any good fishmonger should make, and amounts to fraud. Press your fishmonger for a precise species name for the fish. If you don't get that, this is a shop to be avoided.

SUPERMARKET WET FISH COUNTERS

Since traditional, top-class fish shops are relatively scarce these days, more and more consumers are buying fish in the supermarket. Many supermarkets don't have wet fish counters and, although there are glowing exceptions, those that do are all too frequently unstimulating, lacklustre affairs. Supermarkets state that their wet fish counters are staffed by trained personnel with all the skills of the traditional, high-street fishmonger. Consumer experience suggests that this is not always the case. In fact, most of the fish on offer is usually sent to the store gutted, cleaned and often pre-filleted, to be sold by weight or by the unit. All that the staff have to do in the main is bag it.

A high proportion of fish sold on supermarket wet fish counters has been previously frozen, so much so that it is tempting to refer to them as 'defrosted-fish counters'. That means that more than any other category of foodstuff, you really need to use your eyes and nose to make an astute selection (see page 51). One positive sign to look for in any wet-fish counter is the presence of locally caught fish, sold with a label detailing its origins. Local fish is likely to come more directly to the store and the supermarket has more control over its freshness than exotic products from further away. More supermarkets are developing local buying policies for fresh fish in order to get more control over quality and cut transport costs.

SUPERMARKET PRE-PACKS

Many supermarkets and food retailers don't have fish counters. Instead, fish is sold in pre-packs, either cut up into portions or, in the case of whole fish, cleaned, scaled and gutted. Some fish are simply filleted, put on trays and shrink-wrapped; others are put inside a sealed, transparent container, in what is known as 'controlled-atmosphere' or 'modified-atmosphere' packaging.

If food is left uncovered, the oxygen component in air brings about a number of reactions. In the case of fish, the fats become rancid and smelly and the flesh darkens, dries out and generally shows signs of deterioration. But by upping the ratio of the other two gases in air, nitrogen and carbon dioxide, and substantially reducing the oxygen, the shelf life of food can be extended for anything from two to five times, depending on the product.

This kind of packaging is used extensively for fresh fish and some packs carry a 'fresh never frozen' label. This is most attractive to consumers, many of whom continue to value fresh rather than frozen fish. It looks good and you can see exactly what you are getting.

For the retailer, the advantages are obvious. Although it costs more to pack fish this way (a price increase that can be passed on to the consumer), the shelf life of fish can be much extended. Controlled-atmosphere packaging can give fish an extra ten days' shelf life before it begins to show signs of deterioration. And it is much easier to control the freshness of fish in packs than defrosted fish sitting in normal air on a wet fish counter. Since this type of packaging is thought to be harmless – only a slight modification of the atmosphere that normally surrounds food – retailers are not obliged to state that they have used it. Most consumers have no idea that such packaging exists and merely assume that the fish is as fresh as it looks.

In theory, this sort of packaging could be used by retailers to give fish an artificial freshness. In practice, most responsible retailers use it only as an additional second precaution against spoilage in fish which is very fresh to start with. Most fish sold this way still has a very short sell-by date.

However, the use of this type of technology to slow decay in food raises the question of what real freshness is. Fresh fish, packaged in this way, is only so because of technological intervention. No one knows if consumers welcome this sort of 'freshness' and nobody has consulted them. A legal requirement to state on the label that controlled-atmosphere storage has been used is overdue and would certainly alert more consumers to the currently invisible use of this technology in food retailing. Fortunately controlled-atmosphere storage is quite easy to spot because of the very thick plastic and the strength of the seal.

FRESH VERSUS FROZEN FISH

The merits of fresh versus frozen fish are hotly debated. Although frozen fish tends to have a poorer reputation than fresh, in taste trials it quite often comes out better.

It is silly to argue that any frozen fish can better the taste of absolutely fresh fish straight from the sea but few of us are able to obtain fish of that quality on a regular basis so the question is, which system delivers the best fish to the consumer?

A lot of fish is harvested in deep-water trawlers far out to sea, where it is stored for up to a week in a chilled hold and not particularly carefully treated. Once landed (anything up to eight days after being caught), it is then passed on through fish processors and an increasingly antiquated system of fish markets and wholesalers. 'Fresh' fish may thus be 10 to 14 days old when it reaches the consumer.

On the other hand, fresh fish can come from what are known as 'close water boats'. Despite the name, these are boats that do go far out to sea, so their catch is not likely to be contaminated by pollution from coastal areas, but only for one to three days at a time. Fresh fish by this route tends to taste much better and the smaller-scale nature of the operation is likely to mean that the fish has been better handled too.

Frozen fish often deserves its bad reputation but much depends on exactly how it has been frozen. Some fish is blast-frozen in its box, which can damage the texture and the eating quality. Other fish is frozen individually, using a more gentle process. The best method is to freeze it on the boat immediately after catching and grading. Fish frozen in this way can taste better than the 'fresh' fish described above. Don't buy frozen fish with 'snow' inside the packet. This shows that the pack (and the fish) has suffered from fluctuations in temperature, and is a sign that it has not been well kept.

The problem for the consumer is that fish tends to be sold in a very anonymous way, with no information about how it has been caught, landed, frozen or transported. This is because, in the main, fish is bought and sold as an undifferentiated commodity. Nobody is given any financial incentive to spend extra resources sustaining or improving the quality of their particular output.

Unfortunately price is the only rough guide to quality. The more carefully handled the fish, the more expensive it is likely to be.

JUDGING THE FRESHNESS OF FISH

Don't be inhibited – use your nose! Smell is the first and most obvious indicator of freshness in any fish. It should smell appetisingly fresh and sweet, with a pleasant sea-spray type of aroma. It should not smell sour, 'fishy', sweaty or like ammonia. Fish that smells of silt, dirty harbours or muddy puddles is not good fish, and any that smells vinegary or high should be rejected. The smell should make you want to eat it. Smell is particularly relevant when it comes to fillets or prepared portions, which offer fewer clues to freshness.

Thereafter, you need to look out for visual clues.

In a whole fish...

- The eyes should be sparkling and clear, not dull, sunken or cloudy.
- The gills (just inside where the head meets the belly) should be dark and blood-red, not grey and dirty-looking or slimy.
- The skin should be sleek, shiny and glistening with a transparent mucus, not dull, matt or stuck on to the flesh below.
- Any scales should be firmly attached.
- When you press the fish quite firmly with a finger it should feel resilient and bounce back, leaving no mark.
- The belly of the fish should be firm and closed, with no sagging innards and bulges.
- There should be no odd marks, spots or blemishes on the skin – these can be a sign of pollution.
- The fish should show no signs of rough handling or damage, such as bruising or blood spots, although the odd one is considered acceptable in a wild fish.

In fillets or portions...

- The fish should have an attractive, translucent appearance, with no discoloured flesh, reddening, bruising or blood clots.
- It should be moist, without any signs of dehydration and the fillets or portions should have an even colour and shading (where it has been skinned).
- Avoid fish that is producing liquid or sitting in liquid – it is either badly frozen or, simply, old.

SMOKED FISH

The basic requirement for all good smoked fish is that it is a lovely, fresh, high-quality fish to begin with. So there are some fish to be avoided for this reason. **Smoked Pacific salmon** is usually cheap, imported North American salmon. There are five different species: chinook, chum, sockeye, pink and coho. Although the chinook in particular is considered to be a very fine fish, most Pacific salmon is exported ready canned or brought over to Europe for smoking, where it has to be frozen for long periods. In practice, it is deeply inferior in eating quality to our own fresh Atlantic salmon.

Smoked rainbow trout is usually farmed and has a poor flavour and texture to start with. **Mackerel** can be excellent when fresh but most of the smoked versions on sale are greasy, over-salted and over-peppered. **Boil-in-the-bag kipper fillets** are the worst sort of kipper, often made with inferior imported fish and regularly dyed (see page 55).

Hot or cold smoked?

Some fish, such as the famous Scottish haddock speciality, **Arbroath Smokies**, are hot smoked. This kind of fish does not keep for long and is best eaten fresh, preferably not refrigerated.

Cold-smoked fish, which is first cured or preserved by either dry-salting or brining, keeps much longer. **Salmon** is the most commonly available smoked fish but **halibut, tuna, swordfish** and many more are also available. **Kippers** are herrings that have been split, brined and cold smoked. **Bloaters** – an East Anglian speciality – are herrings that have been slightly dried before smoking and have had the guts left in, which gives them a slightly stronger, gamy taste.

The style for smoking fish varies widely, as does the taste. Some people prefer a strong, assertive style of smoking, sometimes referred to as a **Highland smoke**, but the current fashion is for a lighter style, called a **London smoke**. This produces blander smoked fish, although the theory is that you can taste the fish better. There is a huge difference in flavour according to the wood or fuel that has been used. **Peat-smoked** fish has a much more pronounced flavour than fish smoked over wood such as oak.

Smoked salmon labelling

Labels on smoked salmon are a real trap for the unwary and you have to study them very carefully indeed to be sure of what you are getting. Even then, labelling may leave many questions unanswered.

Having avoided Pacific salmon (see page 53), it is a good idea to buy salmon that clearly states it has been **smoked where it was caught or harvested**. Most salmon on sale in the UK comes from either Scotland, Ireland, the Shetland Isles or Norway. Irrespective of source, go for fish that has been caught and smoked in the same place. Thus a label that states 'Scottish salmon smoked in Scotland' is preferable to either 'Scottish smoked salmon' or 'Smoked Scottish salmon' because the two processes may have been separated: either imports smoked in Scotland or Scottish salmon but smoked elsewhere.

Increasingly, salmon smokers are including a **catching date** and a **smoking date**. Others are adding a **'never frozen'** guarantee. These specific guarantees cut down the chances of buying poorer-quality imported fish that has simply been smoked in one of these countries to give it more value, or salmon that has been smoked, then frozen. However, if it is good salmon to start with, some experts believe that freezing it once smoked (providing it is not for too long) does not harm the flavour.

Unless it specifically states that the fish is wild, you can assume it has been farmed. It is up to you whether you want to buy it or not. If you do buy farmed salmon, look out for labels that offer some environmental guarantees about how it has been raised (see page 68).

Salmon is often sold with 'quality marks' on the label which purport to ensure certain standards. These standards are set by the salmon farming industry, in the main. Their purpose is to encourage sales of Scottish salmon in preference to Norwegian, Shetland and even Irish. They don't take into account many other issues that concern consumers, such as environmental impact.

A proliferation of commercial brands copying, but often slightly changing, these industry quality marks has made them extremely confusing. So when you are buying farmed salmon, go for brands that give you the maximum hard information, not bland assurances.

Colourings in smoked fish

Smoked haddock in its routine, industrial form is coloured with yellow food dyes, both natural and synthetic. The process of smoking gives fish a naturally pale golden colour but many smokers like to make it darker by using colourings such as tartrazine and sunset yellow. The argument goes that these colourings are harmless and some consumers expect their smoked fish to look that way. Many kippers, too, are dyed with a colouring known as brown FK.

There have been doubts raised about the safety of all these dyes, spanning everything from allergic reactions in sensitive people to long-term cancer and birth defects. Toxicity aside, these colourings are certainly not beneficial, and are often used to tart up otherwise poor-looking specimens of fish.

Undyed fish is widely available and infinitely preferable. It is quite easy to spot undyed haddock because it lacks the lurid yellow colour. Kippers are not so easy to distinguish, so you need to look out for a listing of the colour on the ingredients label. If you are buying them loose, check with your fishmonger whether they are coloured or not.

DRIED AND CURED FISH

The simplest dried fish available is **salt cod**, which is imported from Portugal and Africa. It is very heavily salted by what is still an artisanal process, and needs to be soaked for at least 12 hours before use.

Gravad lax is not to be confused with smoked salmon. It has simply been cured with salt and fresh dill, not smoked. All the criteria for choosing salmon (see page 54) should be applied when buying it.

Marinated and sweetcure fish, such as herring, can be wonderful to eat. Unfortunately, most commercial versions are crude and unsubtle. The only test is to try them and, of course, read the label in order to avoid any with chemical additions. Because marinated fish contains so much salt and vinegar there should be no need for chemical preservatives.

FISH FINGERS, CAKES, STICKS AND 'FISH MINCE'

Given that the UK is a maritime nation, it is rather surprising that our consumption of fish is so low. Much of the fish bought in the UK is processed in some way, in the form of cakes, fingers, goujons, nuggets, burgers and so on.

Fish fingers are a classic example of what the food industry calls 'adding value' to a product. There is a limit to what you can charge for straightforward wet fish. However, breaded and coated, mulched up and bound together with additives, then re-formed into different shapes, processed fish products yield a wonderful return on ingredient costs.

Tests on leading brands of fish fingers have revealed that it is the rare finger that contains more than 50 per cent fish. Compared weight for weight with wet fish, the fish in these breaded products works out infinitely more expensive than it should, at least twice the price. This could only be justified if it was of the finest quality but, at best, it represents the most basic white fillets available. At worst, it's what the trade calls 'fish mince'.

Fish mince is produced mechanically either by mincing and sieving white fish or by squeezing and scraping the skeletons of fish that have previously been filleted. This produces a fish sludge or paste, with a texture and taste totally inferior to fillets. The texture is both grittier and mushier because some of the cartilage and skin is broken down along with the scraps of flesh, and the colour is not the attractive white of whole fillets. This low-grade fish paste is used in processed fish products.

Products made from fish mince often contain added water in

the form of polyphosphate solution. This is a food additive which helps bind the food and retain water and therefore bulks out the product. And because the taste of fish mince is not a patch on fillets, certain flavour enhancers, such as salt and monosodium glutamate (see page 261) may be added to 'improve' the taste.

'Crab stick' is an imaginative description for fish mince (sometimes also called surimi), bound together with various starches, egg white, sugar, salt, stabilisers, monosodium glutamate, crab flavouring and some crab (if you are lucky!). It is formed into sticks or into larger blocks that can be sliced up like ham. A crab-like hue is provided by an orange colouring such as paprika.

Scampi should be the tail meat of the small lobster called langoustine or Dublin Bay prawn but most breaded scampi is just an upmarket version of fish mince, where broken tail 'bits' are reformed and moulded back into scampi shape. Unless scampi says 'whole tails' somewhere on the packaging, it is reasonable to assume that it is made up of bits.

Fish cakes, as seen in many local fishmonger's, are generally bought in frozen. They are usually a mixture of fish mince (the law states that this should account for a paltry 35 per cent of the total), water, rehydrated potato powder and salt.

Most **breaded coatings** on fish products are based on rusk, which is dried bread. Many contain items such as sugar and colouring (often paprika), too. Some more upmarket brands use 'oven bake' breadcrumb coatings which are more natural, though even some of these contain colouring. Much healthier home-made alternatives include dipping fish in coarse flour, cornmeal, or fresh breadcrumbs.

Selecting the best breaded products

If you want quality fish for yourself or your children, don't waste your time or money on breaded fish products. However, if you feel under pressure to buy them, select ones that:
- state clearly on the label that the fish inside is whole fillets.
- state the species of fish used (e.g. cod fillet).
- have a short ingredients list (fish, breadcrumbs, salt, oil).

Avoid products that put water near the top of the ingredients list or that contain sugar, colourings (natural or otherwise) and flavour enhancers. Products like these are the bottom of the fish barrel.

EXOTIC FISH

Hoki, red snapper, capitaine, parrot fish, rabbit fish, pomfret, red fish and grouper – just some of the 'exotic' fish that are becoming standard gear in many supermarkets and fishmonger's in metropolitan areas.

Fish like these come mainly from warm temperate or tropical waters in Southeast Asia, right down in the southern hemisphere from the Indian Ocean off Africa, or the colder waters of the Southern Ocean off New Zealand and Australia. They have become very attractive to Northern European fish buyers. Our native fish stocks are under pressure from over-fishing and are now subject to strict quotas, while fish from sources such as the Indian Ocean are relatively plentiful and therefore cheap. Even allowing for air-freight costs, they have become a very attractive business proposition.

Should we be rejoicing? Probably not. However stunning that colourful parrot fish might look, it won't be a patch on native fish from colder, more local waters. Problem number one is that much of this fish seems to be pretty crudely frozen, and the flavour and texture lose a lot in the process. Problem number two is that many of these newly discovered 'exotic' species just aren't so tasty to start with. The main reason we have become interested in them is because our own native fish stocks are more problematic.

However, warm, tropical waters are a good source of shrimps, prawns and large fish such as tuna, and there is some evidence that the increased activity of the European fleet and other huge fishing fleets is having a negative impact on these valuable stocks. Countries such as India, Senegal, Mauritius and Angola, which have ideal coastlines for fishing, are strapped for cash and too inclined to accept fishery 'agreements' with foreign fleets because they need the money.

Multinational fishing companies are being granted fishing licences that entitle them to export their entire catch in return for a tiny percentage of earnings. This sort of deal displaces local fishing boats and often deprives local people of a cheap source of protein. Foreign fleets may fish an area until they have exhausted it, then move on. Local fishers inherit the problems they leave in their wake.

A shortage of fishery protection vessels in such countries makes them particularly vulnerable to boats that do not respect fishing protocols such as exclusion zones. Southern waters are still a relatively untapped source of fish. But environmentalists ask, for how much longer?

THE TRACEABILITY OF TUNA

Where does tuna come from and how is it caught? A simple question, but the answer is not so straightforward. Tuna fishing caused controversy when environmentalists drew attention to the fact that many Pacific yellowfin tuna were being caught in 'wall-of-death' drift nets which, in the process of scooping the tuna from the sea, also killed and damaged other sea creatures such as dolphins. This spawned a number of labels on tinned tuna stating that the fish was caught by environmentally friendly 'pole and line' or 'long line' methods. Such brands use labels such as 'caught with pole and line' to distinguish themselves.

With the exception of Mediterranean and Atlantic tuna, which is usually sold fresh in any case, it is very difficult to be absolutely sure about the origins of tuna once tinned. This is because tuna is often canned in a different country from where it has been fished.

> Tuna fished off the Maldives, Malaysia or Mauritius may have been caught by the local fishing fleet using more artisanal methods or by larger commercial fleets from Japan, South Korea and Taiwan, which look for huge catches by tracing them with sophisticated radar and echo sounders, then encircle them with drift nets. Much of it is sold frozen on the world commodity market, then sent to another country, such as Thailand, for processing and canning. This entitles it to be sold as 'Product of Thailand'.
>
> With such a long and convoluted supply chain, and no comprehensive, independent inspection system, it is very difficult to be sure that tuna has been fished by environmentally friendly methods, and 'dolphin-friendly' claims should be treated with cynicism. Tuna packed and processed where it was fished it likely to represent the catch of the local fleet and, at the very least, has provided income and jobs for people there.

FRESHWATER FISH

With the exception of trout farmed in rivers and salmon, which is both a freshwater and saltwater fish, freshwater fish has all but disappeared from the fishmonger's slab. Species such as carp, pike, whitefish, perch and eel used to be found in rivers and lakes in relative abundance but the progressive build-up of toxins in rivers, reservoirs and waterways has put paid to that. Most freshwater fish are now caught for sport, not food, and anglers tend to return them to the river.

Freshwater fish is variable in taste and texture and rarely matches the flavour of saltwater fish. It can, however, be quite fine and delicious but you have to be absolutely certain about the source. Brown trout from a remote Scottish or Irish stream can be clean and exquisite, but in areas of industry and near large centres of population freshwater fish is likely to give you a concentrated shot of whatever nasties are around. Don't eat this type of fish unless you trust the source absolutely. Never buy freshwater fish of anonymous origins – fish that has been poached or 'fallen off the back of a lorry'. Poachers use very nasty chemicals that can poison salmon pools to help them catch fish. Imported freshwater fish have probably been frozen first and there is no guarantee that they are any cleaner than fish caught in Britain.

Farmed fish

More and more of the fish on sale these days is farmed. As natural stocks of fish have declined (see page 42), so fish farming has boomed. Aquaculture, as it is also known, has been carried out throughout the world in fairly small-scale forms for thousands of years, but since the 1960s it has become big business. Aquaculture now produces 20 per cent of the global total of fish consumed. Unfortunately, it is rapidly becoming the factory farming of the sea, increasingly owned and controlled by large transnational companies.

Fish farming has changed our supply of fish out of all recognition. Previously seasonal fish such as salmon are now available fresh all year round, at a fraction of the former price. Rainbow trout are as ubiquitous as ice in the fishmonger's window, despite the fact that they are consistently flaccid, watery travesties of what was once a fine, athletic fish.

As farmed salmon and trout have become everyday and unexceptional, fish farmers have moved on to other species. Fish such as turbot, bream, bass, halibut and Arctic char – previously only available in the wild – are now being farmed. Some freshwater species, such as the Mississippi catfish, are being farmed in the USA and imported here. Prawn farming is big business in Asia and tropical Latin America.

In theory, fish farming is a clever idea. Demarcate an area of water, stock it with fish in large underwater cages, feed them food that is the equivalent of what they would eat in the wild and then harvest them when they reach the appropriate weight. The marine equivalent of having your cake and eating it, it allows farmers to exploit natural resources without having to put up with the infamous capriciousness of Nature. Fish farming offers tantalising promise – a regular marine harvest and a steady supply for the consumer.

There is a big commercial bonus for the fish farmers, too. Fish farming can make good business sense because it also gives a much more standard catch – no small fish mixed up with whoppers. The farmer can rear and sort out all fish at a similar weight. Smaller fish are attractive to many consumers because they cost less per fish, even though the price per pound is the same.

Unfortunately, although there are a few systems for farming salmon that are vastly superior to the standard approach (see page 67), most farmed fish, like factory-farm animals, spend their lives in an artificial environment that is alien to their natural behaviour patterns. The result, all too often, is a sadly debased foodstuff, with chronic environmental problems in formerly unspoiled coastal regions and question marks over the implications for human health.

THE QUALITY OF FARMED FISH

The fish-farming industry has put a lot of time and effort into persuading consumers that there is little or no difference in quality between farmed and wild fish. They have met with only partial success. In the USA, farmed fish is regarded as better than wild, which is suspect because of sea and river pollution. Amongst chefs and food lovers in Europe, however, farmed fish has a poor image, although some farmed fish is better than others (see page 67). Advocates of fish farming put this preference for wild fish down to snobbery. For the average consumer, the usual price advantage of farmed over wild, plus the difficulty in obtaining wild fish, has brought acceptance of the products of fish farming, albeit with reservations. Only an estimated 2 per cent of salmon caught in the UK is wild.

You cannot always assume that wild fish is the best bet. Wild salmon, for example, is often badly handled, caught in tangle nets or fish traps, and not put on ice until several hours after catching, while farmed is generally better handled. However, there is no doubt that wild fish caught at the right time and handled properly afterwards has an incomparable flavour. Taste trials have shown that there are quite perceptible differences between wild and farmed fish.

- **Texture:** Farmed fish tend to have wetter flesh which dries out rapidly during cooking, while wild fish are initially firmer and remain more juicy.
- **Flabbiness:** Tests show that farmed fish are significantly fattier than their wild equivalents (up to ten times fattier for certain fish). Often farmed fish give off water in cooking.
- **Smell:** Wild fish smell sweet while farmed fish can smell a bit muddy (although wild fish can taste like this when harvested too late because sexual maturation is underway).
- **Taste:** Farmed fish tend to taste neutral. Different species, such as bass and bream, may be impossible to tell apart when tasted blind. Wild fish, on the other hand, seem to retain flavours inherent to their particular species.

These differences between farmed and wild fish are a direct consequence of the contrasts in their lifestyles – as stark as the differences between a factory-farm pig and a wild boar.

Lack of exercise

Fish are athletic creatures, who can swim for thousands of miles in the wild. Under modern farming conditions they are kept in drastically restricted circumstances and their natural instinct to exercise properly is severely limited. At certain points in their life cycle, farmed fish can be confined 50 at a time in one cubic metre of water. Like lazy, cooped-up humans, they become fatter and flabbier.

A uniform diet...

Farmed fish are fed on pellets – artificial food designed to mimic the diet they would normally find in the wild. These are small fish, algae and crustaceans at the bottom of the marine food chain, although recycled dead fish from fish farms can also be processed into pellets. All species of farmed fish are fed the same diet, irrespective of the fact that different species would seek out different feeding in the wild. The pellets and granules used in modern fish farming mainly contain meal made from mulched-up 'industrial' fish, such as sand eel, sprat, capelin, krill and Norway pout. These are species that have been over-fished in waters such as the North Sea, and stocks of them are under pressure. The biggest customer for fish meal is not, in fact, aquaculture, but agriculture, since it is widely used in livestock feed, too. Whether fed to fish or animals, fish meal is rich in protein. Combined with added vitamins, these feeds have the effect of accelerating growth. Though some wild fish who find really good feeding grounds can grow very fast, farmed fish generally reach their desirable weight faster, thus giving the farmer a quicker return on investment. Farmed trout, for example, can reach maturity in nine months, whereas in the wild, it might take 13 to 18 months.

...With a few added extras

Fish kept in such unnaturally confined conditions are prone to a variety of diseases and infestations by parasites such as sea lice (see below), which affect their health and appearance. This means that they have to be medicated routinely. Antibiotics are usually mixed in with the pellet feed by the company that supplies it, although this practice is giving way to the vaccination of fish.

Artificial colours are added to the feed of salmon and trout to make it pink, whereas wild equivalents pick up this colour naturally from the crustaceans on which they feed. The most commonly used colouring is Canthaxanthin – a chemical substance that has been pinpointed as being toxic and is not recommended for use in foods. Many fish farm companies switched to another similar chemical colouring, Astaxanthin, which is said to be less toxic, then reverted to Canthaxanthin because they could not produce the depth of colour deemed necessary in the time available.

Cleaning up farmed fish

Intensive farming of fish in overcrowded conditions produces a problem – sea lice. In the wild, a salmon, for example, would normally lose any lice as it entered freshwater on migration. Fish in cages cannot do this, and so sea lice has become a major affliction, which can cause high mortality rates.

The standard way to treat it is by bathing the fish in a dilute solution of an extremely toxic chemical and marine pesticide called Dichlorvos. Because this is only effective against the adult stage of the louse, the fish have to be treated once and then again ten days later. So salmon stocks are often treated with it several times a year. It takes quite some time to treat a whole site, so the lice can migrate from treated to untreated pens and nullify the treatment. Some farmers get on to a treadmill of repeated treating which can result in a permanent presence of low levels of Dichlorvos throughout an entire loch.

Dichlorvos is on the government's Red List of most dangerous substances and is known to be devastating to other marine life, even at very weak concentrations. Experiments have been made to find alternatives to Dichlorvos, including using small seafish – wrasse – who like to eat sea lice. But wrasse get lice too, so they are not a foolproof solution. This sort of natural predator approach is not at all widespread in fish farming. Hydrogen peroxide has been found to work but it is very expensive and so not commonly used.

In addition, other disinfectants, fungicides, algicides and pesticides are used for cleaning cages and preventing weed build-up on nets.

EFFECTS OF FISH FARMING ON HUMAN HEALTH

The apparently routine medication of farmed fish has worrying implications for human health. Several of the antibiotics used routinely in aquaculture are also used in human medicine. There is a strong possibility that these antibiotics could be made less effective, or even totally useless, by resistance passed on from farmed fish. Certain diseases amongst farmed fish are already proving resistant to some commonly used antibiotics.

When fish have been treated with medicines, producers are meant to observe strict 'withdrawal' periods, so that all traces of the medicine have disappeared before the fish is put on sale. But spot checks on farmed salmon have shown that this is not always the case. Residues of highly toxic Dichlorvos have been found in farmed salmon. 'Malachite green', a potentially teratogenic (producing malformation in the foetus) and carcinogenic coal tar dye used as a fungicide, has been found contaminating over 10 per cent of samples in government spot checks, as has Ivermectin, an animal medicine whose use in fish is illegal.

IMPACT OF FISH FARMING ON THE ENVIRONMENT

Keeping huge numbers of fish concentrated in a tiny area has serious consequences for the surrounding environment. Fish wastes, excess feed and chemicals used for cleaning up and de-lousing all contribute to water pollution. Solid waste from fish farms forms a silt below the cages and this contributes to a reduction in water oxygen levels. Soluble waste adds unwanted nutrients to the water, increasing the incidence of algal blooms, which can be highly toxic to fish and marine life.

Since the mid-1980s there has been an alarming decline in the numbers of wild salmon and sea trout being caught, and there is evidence that sea lice, spread from fish farms by escaping fish, has infected wild stocks. There is also concern that escapee farmed fish, no longer programmed for existing in the wild, are breeding with wild stock. This may produce offspring with a reduced ability to cope in the natural environment and lead to a long-term diminution in wild stocks.

Other wildlife such as otters have been shot at fish farms, where they are considered to be pests. Seabirds, dolphins, basking sharks and porpoises can all be caught in the 'anti-predator' nets employed by fish farms.

WELFARE OF FARMED FISH

In the wild, species such as salmon spend most of their adult life roaming the seas. When they are farmed their natural instincts are totally inhibited because they are kept in relatively small floating cages or pens, usually made of nylon bag nets, suspended on a frame of steel or plastic. Animal welfarists, using a relatively low stocking density rate of 15 kilos of fish per cubic metre, calculate that this is like keeping a half-metre-long salmon in a bathtub of water. In Scotland, a typical stocking density is even greater, at around 20–25 kilos, while in Norway it can be as much as 30 kilos or more. There are no regulations governing how farmed fish should be killed. It is thought that many simply suffocate slowly when they are taken out of the water, taking up to 15 minutes to lose consciousness. More compassionate farmers replace the oxygen in water with carbon dioxide, which quickly kills the fish, or use electrocution or a short club known as a 'priest', which kills instantly when properly used.

IMPROVING FISH FARMING

In response to widespread criticism, a number of farmers in Ireland and Scotland are trying new approaches which take into account the welfare of the fish and the impact on the environment. Some salmon farmers are trying extensive fishing, which involves rearing their fish in much larger pens further out at sea, where there are stronger tides. The tides keep the sites clear of any build-up of seabed detritus and give the fish the exercise they need. There is also less chance of pollution from effluent because the fish are more dispersed, further away from the mouths of rivers and coastline.

In these superior systems, fewer salmon are kept in each pen. This means more swimming space, so the fish have much firmer flesh. Feeds are often made up to order to ensure that only good-quality fish meal is used. It has been shown that routine medication of fish feed can be done away with and that chemicals to disinfect and clean up are not necessary. Natural pest-control methods, such as using wrasse to control lice and dummy sharks to scare away erstwhile predators like otters and seals, are all being tried out, often with encouraging results.

Fish produced under these less intensive conditions are likely to taste better than standard farmed fish and have a pleasingly firm flesh, akin to wild salmon. They also cost significantly more. The extensive fish farmer does not benefit from the same economies of scale as one who rears the maximum number of fish in the small-est possible area, and so cut-throat is the competition between rival fish farmers that price cutting is the name of the game. Not a situation likely to lead to an emphasis on the overall healthiness and quality of farmed fish.

HOW TO DISTINGUISH FARMED FISH FROM WILD

There is no legal obligation for fish retailers to state whether a fish is farmed or wild. This is a serious omission, since the knowledge that a fish is wild is the best guarantee that it will taste good.

In the case of salmon and trout you can assume that it is farmed unless it is specifically labelled otherwise. If the label says wild, it is reasonable to expect that your fishmonger can tell you the source of the fish and how he or she knows that it is wild. Frauds are common!

Ultimately, buying fish is a matter of trust. Well-respected fish-mongers have a lot to lose by trying to pass off farmed fish as wild, since the difference between the two fish, even visually, is usually apparent to anyone with a slight knowledge of fish. Wild salmon, for example, have spikier, less even-looking dorsal and tail fins than farmed ones, which tend to be more rounded.

With newly commercialised species of fish – 'prime' fish such as bass, bream, turbot or halibut – the difference may be less obvious. Again, ask your fishmonger about the source of the fish, and watch out for fish of an even size becoming a standard feature of the display – they are probably farmed. Wild fish come and go fleetingly, dependent on storms at sea, fishing stocks and so on, and they will vary in size. Prime wild fish do not come in by standard weight, neither are they an everyday occurrence!

IDENTIFYING BETTER-QUALITY FARMED SALMON

More naturally reared farmed salmon are relatively few and far between but are becoming increasingly popular. They are usually retailed with explanatory leaflets and packaging that gives you information about production methods, and are most likely to be found in good independent fishmonger's. Some large retailers do stock this kind of salmon but the difference may not be explicit on the labelling, since they do not want consumers to think that, by implication, there is something less desirable about their standard farmed fish. Certain 'prime' salmon labels may be more environmentally sound farmed fish – but the only way you can know that is by writing to the chain and asking!

Selecting shellfish

There is nothing quite like a huge plate of shellfish, stacked up on glistening ice and surrounded by wedges of fresh lemon. Shellfish has a marvellous celebratory feel. It is a real 'hands-on' food, which encourages people to be uninhibited and sociable.

When shellfish is in fine condition it can leave you feeling exhilarated and somewhat restored. This is because raw seafood, particularly oysters, is a great source of important trace elements such as zinc, which are often lacking in modern diets. Aphrodisiac qualities may be an exaggeration but there is no doubt that a meal of fresh, clean seafood can really perk you up.

Clean, however, is the operative word. Bad or contaminated raw shellfish can make you very ill indeed and even kill you. There are enough cases of shellfish-related food poisoning every year to put it in the risky food category.

Different types of seafood don't carry the same risks. Shellfish is a ragbag term which can be broken down into two groups.

The first group is **crustaceans**, such as crab, lobster, shrimps, prawns and langoustines. These tend to come from relatively unpolluted waters far from shore and are therefore less prone to contamination. In addition, they are eaten cooked, cutting down the risk of bacterial contamination. All in all, they are pretty safe to eat. The same cannot be said for the second group, **molluscs**. These have shells and are divided into two sub-types: **univalves**, such as winkles and whelks, have only one shell, while **bivalves**, such as oysters, mussels, cockles, clams and scallops have two shells hinged together.

Bivalve molluscs are particularly prone to contamination because of the way they feed, which means they accumulate micro-organisms in their body. So if there is a nasty virus or bacterial infection around they are likely to contain a concentrated dose of it. This risk applies mainly to molluscs that grow near-shore or in estuaries, because it is common practice to pump untreated sewage and industrial waste into the sea at precisely such points. (This does not apply to scallops, which are harvested much further out to sea.)

Near-shore molluscs are dredged up and then have to be purged to 'render them fit for human consumption' before they can be sold. This can be done by putting them into tanks of pure water, which is irradiated with ultra-violet light. They are there just long enough to allow them to rid themselves of the offending organisms.

Alternatively, the molluscs can be moved into an area of clean water until they purify themselves. Even then they are not exactly clean, because while these treatments remove bacterial contamination they cannot shift viruses or remove pollutants such as pesticides, heavy metals and other toxins. Even if they are not contaminated with anything actively nasty, they tend to be dirty, sandy and covered in barnacles, with many broken shells. This is because they have been dredged up and subsequently handled rather a lot.

All this means that for anyone who is pregnant, has a weakened immune system or simply doesn't fancy taking a risk, even 'purified' molluscs are off-limits. Grill your fishmonger or supermarket as to the geographical source of the molluscs before you buy them. If they come from the Wash, North Wales or Holland, avoid them. Buy 'cultured' alternatives from clean water instead (see below).

Never eat molluscs that you have harvested yourself.

CULTURED SHELLFISH

One welcome development in aquaculture is that certain otherwise risky bivalve molluscs, such as mussels and oysters, can now be cultivated.

Many **mussels** available these days are produced by what is known as 'hanging culture', or 'rope-grown'. Ropes are hung from rafts in the sea, the mussels attach themselves to the ropes and grow to maturity feeding naturally by extracting plankton from the sea.

This type of mussel culture works only in areas where the sea is still clean. The finest cultured mussels come from the West Highlands, the Outer Hebrides and the West and South of Ireland. Mussels grown in this way are highly unlikely to be contaminated, though they are regularly tested. They do not need to be purified because they are naturally clean to start with.

As well as being clean and uncontaminated, rope-grown

mussels tend to be free of dirt and sand, since this is not part of their environment, and they have smooth, fine shells. Because they are rope-grown, harvesting is easy, so they have a much better chance of reaching the shops with their shells intact.

Rope-culture mussels are excellent to eat and very safe. They are generally inexpensive to buy, though they do cost more than the less desirable dredged, near-shore type. Most fishmongers label rope-cultured mussels as such, or at the very least can tell you whether they are or not. It is relatively easy to tell the difference between cultured and dredged mussels because the former are usually very clean, free of grit, smooth and shiny. The latter often look dirty, dull and gritty and as though someone has danced a Highland jig on them. Happily, cultured mussels are the most common type available in British shops these days.

Cultivated **scallops** are grown in nets suspended in water in the same type of environment as cultivated mussels. Scallops that have not been cultivated are usually caught by divers to avoid grit. Scallops can be dredged but they end up dirty and unattractive, and therefore have a lower value. Most scallops, either cultivated or diver-caught, are of a high quality and clean.

Oysters used to be a food for the masses. However, disease and pollution put paid to most of our 'native' or indigenous oyster beds which were home to the species, *Ostrea edulis*. Native oysters are now few and far between. Most oysters you see in the shops are cultivated and a different variety, *Crassotrea gigas*, better known as the Pacific oyster.

These oysters are cultivated in suitable water around the British Isles. Oyster larvae, or 'spat', are encouraged to attach themselves to specially placed supports inside special collector areas below the water. Like rope-grown mussels, they feed naturally on plankton from the water. The best ones come from the west coast, Ireland and the North of Scotland, where they are cultivated in sea lochs. Because the water there is very clean they do not need to be purified before they are sold. However, some Pacific oysters, cultivated in sea estuaries and along east-coast areas, are more prone to pollution, so they do have to be transferred into clean, purified water for a period before sale. Always ask about the precise geographical origins of oysters before you buy them.

Oysters are usually sold by unit price and have a luxury image. Since six oysters is usually enough to serve one, they represent a very high-quality, nutritious food at a relatively low price.

JUDGING THE FRESHNESS OF RAW SHELLFISH

Crustaceans
- They should smell fresh and sweet.
- They should glisten with moisture.
- Legs, heads, pincers and tails should never be loose or detached from the body. Preferably, they should still be moving.

Molluscs
- Shells should look smooth and shiny and only a tiny proportion (two or three per kilo) should be broken or damaged.
- There should be no signs of dirt, mud or silt.
- In bivalves, the shells should be tightly shut. The few that are open should clam up when the flesh inside is gently touched with the blade of a knife. Never eat any that don't close after being touched. (The only exception are scallops, which do not need to be alive when cooked.)
- Oysters should feel heavy in the hand.

And when there's an 'r' in the month…?

There is still some common sense to the old maxim, 'Never eat oysters unless there is an "r" in the month.' Although cultivated bivalves may be available on a year-round basis, the summer months, especially May and June, are the high-risk times for bivalve contamination. This is when water (mainly east coast) is most likely to be affected by 'red tides', a sort of algal bloom on the surface of water.

There is a debate over whether this is a natural phenomenon or encouraged by pollution. Either way, it can make bivalves extremely poisonous. Though this sort of problem is very rare in most areas where shellfish is cultivated, many people prefer to eat bivalves only in the cooler months (see page 76).

PRE-COOKED SHELLFISH

Only buy cooked shellfish, such as prawns, lobster and langoustines, if you are very sure of your source, because it is much more difficult to judge their freshness. Cooking pre-cooked crustaceans again is a waste of time and money, because the poor things will have no flavour at all. Most cooked crustaceans will have been cooked from frozen, although this will probably not be stated on the label, and many consumers would prefer ones cooked fresh, given the choice. Amongst ready-cooked crustaceans, those with the shell left on seem to retain more flavour, mainly because they have not been shelled in water first (see page 75). Avoid those with white-looking shells – a sign of dehydration. Molluscs overcook easily and do not lend themselves to reheating, so most are sold raw.

Tinned or bottled shellfish in brine or vinegar bears no resemblance to its raw self and is to be avoided.

SMOKED SHELLFISH

Smoked shellfish is becoming more commonly available. Certain bivalves, such as mussels, oysters, queen scallops and razor clams, are now sold smoked on the half shell. These can be delicious but poor-quality ones are over-salty and rubbery, something you cannot tell until you taste them. They are already 'cooked' by the smoke and do not need any further cooking.

FROZEN SHELLFISH

While you can argue the toss over the relative merits of fresh and frozen fish, frozen shellfish *never* compares favourably with fresh.

Certain bivalves, such as scallops, their diminutive siblings quee-nies, and all kinds of clams are particularly damaged by freezing. This manifests itself in a rubberiness when cooked and a rapid loss of water. Prawns and shrimps of all kinds support freezing rather better, though even the best are second best to fresh. Almost more than with fresh shellfish, you have to buy the most expensive upmarket brands to get something worth eating. Even then, by the time they have been processed they probably won't taste of very much.

This is because most frozen prawns are usually bought fresh, then frozen in the shell by a processor. They are then shelled by removing the head and holding the tail in front of a very power-ful jet of water to force the meat out of the shell. During this process they collect quite a lot of water which is then frozen in with the prawn again. Most frozen prawns have thus been frozen twice by the time you buy them. The poorest frozen prawns are to be had in the form of 'scampi', which has become a name for broken bits of prawn tail, bound together with polyphosphates and some 'fish mince', 're-formed' into prawn shape and dipped in batter and breadcrumbs.

As a rule, frozen raw prawns are always better than frozen cooked ones, which are often overcooked and entirely tasteless. In the main, the bigger the prawn the better. Indian Ocean flower and tiger prawns, farmed from warm tropical waters, seem to be meaty enough to stand up to freezing reasonably well. They fare rather better than the theoretically more flavoursome cold-water prawns fished off countries such as Norway, Greenland and Iceland. These often have large amounts of salt poured on to give them some taste.

Cheaper brands of frozen prawns are a rip-off. These are often 'ice-glazed' when they are frozen and have water added to reduce the natural drying out that would otherwise occur when they are defrosted. Tests have shown that all brands of frozen prawns con-tain water but this varies from 10 to 50 per cent of the weight of the prawns. The seemingly cheaper brands often work out more expensive in the end when this is taken into account. So, when buying frozen prawns, only buy those that state the weight of prawns, *exclusive* of glaze. The label should say either 'deglazed weight', 'after defrosting', 'net of ice glaze' or 'weight before protective ice glaze added'.

The labelling of frozen shellfish is very inadequate. It is common for prawns to be frozen after they are caught, held in store, defrosted to process and then frozen again. The fresh (unfrozen) prawns you buy could have been frozen first. They could be cooked, then frozen, or frozen, then cooked and frozen again . . . and that's just the legal treatment, not allowing for any small-time fraud! When you buy prawns far from their harvesting source there is no way you can really be sure of what you are getting.

Fish and shellfish seasons

It may not be obvious from looking at the fishmonger's slab, but fish and shellfish, like fruit and vegetables, do have seasons. While fish displays may rely on a year-round supply of items such as farmed salmon, imported exotic fish and cultivated mussels, many of our standard fish are not so obliging. The main time to avoid is the spawning season, which varies from species to species. At this time the flesh softens and the taste is disappointing. Bivalve shellfish like mussels may offer little eating, while oysters can become too 'milky'. At other times in the year, certain species migrate as water temperatures change, so they may become unavailable, except for frozen.

The chart below shows the optimum season for the most commonly consumed fish and shellfish and the months when they are best avoided or are unavailable. In months not mentioned, the item may be on sale but the eating quality will not be at its best.

Type	Best Season	Avoid/Unavailable
Brill	January–March	May–August
Cockles	All year	–
Cod	January, February, September–December	March–April
Coley	January, February, September–December	–
Crab	April–June	January–March
Dover sole	June–February	March, April
Eel	October–December	May–August
Flounder	January–March	April–June
Grey mullet	July–February	March–June
Haddock	May–February	March, April
Hake	June–February	March–May
Halibut	July–April	May, June
Herring	June–February	April
Huss (dogfish)	October–March	June–August
John Dory	January–March	April–December
Langoustine (Dublin Bay prawn, scampi)	All year	–
Lemon sole	December–April	May, June
Ling	September–February	–
Lobster	April–September	January–March
Mackerel	November–June	–
Monkfish	All year	–
Mussels	September–December, March–May	–
Oysters	September–April	–
Pilchards	August–October	Rest of year
Plaice	July–December	February–April

The Food We Eat

Type	Best Season	Avoid/Unavailable
Prawns	May–October	–
Red mullet	July–September	October–April
Salmon (Wild)	April–August	September–January
Sardines	June–August	September–February
Scallops and Queenies	December–March	–
Sea bass/bream	June–December	Rest of year
Sea trout	March–July	Rest of year
Shrimps	March–October	–
Skate	September–February	–
Sprats	October–March	Rest of year
Squid	May–October	–
Tuna	All year	–
Turbot	August–February	–
Whitebait	February–July	Rest of year
Whiting	November–February	–
Witch sole	August–April	Rest of year

Chicken, Turkey and Other Farmed Poultry

When you are buying poultry it is worth remembering that the eating quality of any bird depends on three factors: the breed, a wholesome diet and plentiful exercise. This applies every bit as much to farmed birds as it does to wild.

The birds should come from breeds developed for flavour and they should spend most of their daytime out of doors, pecking at good, natural vegetation in the earth which is then supplemented by balanced 'rations' fed by the farmer. A decent feed should consist overwhelmingly of grain, with other natural foodstuffs such as dried grass and seaweed which are rich in natural vitamins, minerals and trace elements.

A diet like this, combined with regular exercise and the ability to satisfy certain basic instincts – dustbathing, perching, making nests, flying and so on – produces birds that are delicious to eat and whose welfare is assured into the bargain.

Too little British poultry fits the bill. Most of what we see for sale is reared in factory farms, where fast-growing modern breeds are treated as units of production in a drive to turn out the maximum amount of cheap meat in the shortest possible time. It is a pretty unrewarding and joyless transaction all round. The birds have miserable lives and we get tasteless, characterless meat.

Consumers are finally getting fed up with this and many more free-range birds are becoming available. A 'free-range' tag does not necessarily offer the reassurance about animal welfare or food safety that many consumers seek (see page 87) but most are an improvement on standard British poultry.

If you want flavoursome poultry that has been humanely raised you will need to be prepared to pay more for it. A chicken, turkey or duck that fits the bill will price itself as a weekly treat, but that outlay should be more than compensated for by its radically superior eating qualities.

The 'standard' table bird

If you buy basic table poultry – sold simply as 'fresh', 'farm', 'British' or some equally meaningless title – it is salutary to remember exactly what you are getting. **Broiler chickens** (as chickens for eating rather than egg laying are known) spend their unnaturally short lives (42 days) shut up in sheds, packed so closely that by the time they reach maturity, they have less space to sit on than a telephone directory. They are from modern strains of poultry that have been bred not for their flavour but for their ability to put on a significant amount of weight in a short time. **Poussins**, or **spring chickens**, are less mature broilers that are killed at around 28 days. (The natural lifespan of a chicken is anything from five to ten years.)

Chicks are put on top of litter, usually a deep layer of woodshavings. Because the birds are so tightly packed it is not feasible to change this litter again until the shed is emptied for slaughter. By the time a broiler has reached its slaughter weight, the litter stinks and is caked with droppings and any spills from the automated feeding lines and water drinkers.

Kept in these barren and frustrating circumstances, chickens suffer. Many develop deformed feet. Selective breeding means that their leg muscles cannot keep up with the weight of their breasts. Because they have to scramble over the caked litter to get to food and water points, they develop burns on their breasts and legs from lying on it. There are higher than average rates of heart disease, fatty livers and kidneys. Sickly birds may even die in amongst the litter without the stockperson noticing, because the litter is literally 'carpeted' with birds. In hot weather especially, mortality is particularly high (more than the regular 6 per cent), and many birds die from dehydration and stress.

At the end of their miserable existence the birds are caught and put into crates for slaughter. In such cramped circumstances, this often means rough handling. The birds are not strong to start with and their bones are weak from lack of exercise. Selective breeding for plump breasts means that broilers are top heavy and their frame is supporting a far greater weight of flesh than it ought to, predisposing the birds to leg weakness. As a result, many broilers have dislocated hips and suffer other injuries before final slaughter.

WHAT BROILER CHICKENS CAN EAT

The feed of broiler chickens is very unlikely to be of the best quality because of the pressure on farmers to produce meat cheaply. The standard grain-based diet can quite legally be supplemented with high-protein foods, such as soya, which accelerate the growth rate. Less savoury and much cheaper protein additions can quite legally include other animal and fish protein wastes.

Because disease is rife in broiler systems, medicated feed containing antibiotics and other preventative drugs can be routinely added to the standard feed to prevent outbreaks that might slow down growth.

Turkeys, ducks, guinea fowl and quail

Turkeys live longer than broilers (12 to 26 weeks), though their natural lifespan is around 10 years. They are kept either in 'pole barns', which may have some fresh air and light through chicken wire, or indoor 'compounds', 'yards', 'verandah' and 'wire cage' systems — the turkey equivalent of broiler houses. Either way, they are extremely densely packed and proper exercise is impossible. There is no legal upper limit on the number of turkeys that can be kept in one shed. Large units can house as many as 10,000.

Turkeys are semi-wild birds, more like pheasants than chicken, and it is only since the 1960s that they have been reared indoors. This means that they are less passive, and more likely to react against their unnatural circumstances by attacking each other. For this reason, turkey chicks have their beak tips cut off routinely with a red-hot blade — a mutilation which is known to cause chronic long-term suffering.

Turkeys eat a similar diet to broiler chickens and, because disease is every bit as common, antibiotics and other animal medicines in feed are standard practice. The mortality rate is 7 per cent.

Even more so than broiler chickens, turkeys suffer badly from being bred to have an unnaturally large amount of breast meat. This predisposes them to leg injuries and lameness as their frames simply cannot carry the weight. They are also too top-heavy to mate with each other naturally, so the females have to be artificially inseminated by methods that are unpleasant, for both the birds and the stockperson.

There is a lot of evidence to suggest that turkeys often end their lives in great pain and distress. These very heavy birds are shackled by their legs to a slowly moving slaughtering line. Quite legally, they can hang like that for up to six minutes.

The **ducks, guinea fowl and quail** you see widely on sale are likely to come from specialised intensive poultry farms, where their lives are every bit as unfortunate as those of broiler chickens and turkeys, although ducks and guinea fowl are given more space and generally kept in smaller groups. Some imported birds in these categories are raised in slightly better circumstances, with more space, a better diet, room to nest and perch and so on. But unless such refinements are explicitly stated on the label, assume that they are not.

JUDGING THE QUALITY OF CHICKEN

The best breeds of chicken, such as the **Cou nu**, **Rock Cornish** and **Bresse** (see below), look different from the standard modern broiler. They have higher, narrower breasts, more like pheasants, and large, strong legs from outdoor exercise. There is a distinct difference in colour between the paler breast meat and the legs, which are much darker. The carcass should look nice and smooth with no marks, bruises or blood spots – a sign of rough handling when caught. There should be no spots or pimples, since these are indicators of disease. The chicken should smell clean and neutral with no off-odours. Chicken brought fresh, not frozen, which contains or exudes a lot of water, has been wet-plucked, and water has been retained in the bird. This is not a very good sign for overall quality. Though most birds are wet-plucked, they should not end up watery. Take it back to the shop. Dry-plucked birds are found in top butcher's and supermarkets, but usually only at Christmas.

THE QUALITY OF PRE-PORTIONED POULTRY

Chicken wings, turkey legs, duck breasts … any kind of pre-portioned poultry will have come from an intensive system *unless the label explicitly states otherwise*. Only a small amount of pre-portioned poultry available in up-market shops and supermarket branches is from birds that qualify for the basic 'free-range' tag (see page 87). So if you want better-tasting, more welfare-conscious poultry, buy whole birds.

READY-BASTED OR BUTTER-BASTED BIRDS

These are birds, usually turkeys, that have been injected with ingredients such as butter, vegetable oil, salt, sugar, lactose, synthetic flavourings, hydrolised vegetable protein and stock to make them tender. This injection is done mechanically, and then the basting medium is massaged into the birds. A decent, tasty bird should not need this type of technological intervention. However, it is becoming more common as a technique to render unctuous the dry and tasteless turkey breast meat produced by intensive farming.

Variations on the poultry theme: an at-a-glance guide

CHICKEN (BY AGE AND SEX)

Broiler is just the name given to chickens reared for the table, as opposed to egg-laying hens.

Poussins (spring chickens) are immature chickens. They may appear more tender but are usually reared in an intensive way and so will have little flavour.

Capons are large, neutered male chickens which are specially fattened and allowed to grow much older and therefore heavier than the standard chicken. They have a large amount of white breast meat and are often considered as a good halfway house between chicken and turkey. Free-range capon is likely to have a good flavour but indoor-reared birds will be disappointing.

Boiling hens are usually egg-laying hens whose productiveness has dropped and whose lives are therefore 'uneconomic'. Unless they are free-range or organic, they are best avoided, since they will have spent their lives in a cage or a barn, eating a poor-quality diet. If you can get a free-range or organic bird, the meat will be tough but, for a stock base or soup, the flavour may be wonderful.

Cocks are very old unneutered male birds. If they come out of an intensive system they are likely to have been kept for breeding, and the same objections apply as with boiling hens. Free-range or organic cocks can have an excellent flavour after marinating and long, slow cooking, when they end up tasting more like game birds. Like red meat, cocks need to be hung to make them tender.

CHICKEN (BY BREED AND FEED)

Yellow (maize-fed) chickens have been fed on a diet whose cereal element consists largely of corn. This type of feeding is popular in Southwest France. Maize is thought to give the birds a particularly good flavour but flavour also depends on other factors, such as whether the chicken is free-range, the breed, and so on. You cannot assume automatically that a yellow chicken will taste any better than a white one. However, yellow colouring is a sign that the bird has been fed on a high-quality grain diet rather than pelleted rations.

Cou nu is particularly popular in France. It is an older, more flavoursome breed which takes longer to reach its final weight (minimum 81 days). These birds are more expensive to rear and therefore not adapted to factory farming.

Bresse chickens are deservedly famous birds which are reared in free-range conditions just north of Lyon. Many chefs rate them as having the best flavour of any chicken in the world, due to the combination of traditional rearing skills, high-quality, natural feed and the vegetation in the area, which seems to be particularly suitable for nourishing pecking. Bresse chickens are available only in specialist shops and are extremely expensive.

Landes chickens come from the eponymous area in Southwest France and are often on sale in Britain. They are usually from the Cou nu breed (see above), maize-fed and free-ranging. They have a much better flavour than most British broiler chickens.

The leg meat is much darker and chewier than the breast meat, which means that more careful cooking is required. Landes chickens are found in some supermarkets.

Black-leg chicken is a traditional French breed. As well as having a slightly better flavour than standard white chicken, it has firmer flesh which, though tender, lends itself to longer, slower cooking. They are widely available in supermarkets and good butchers around Christmas but may be hard to find during the rest of the year.

Rock Cornish hen is a slow-growing chicken which thrives outdoors and is more flavoursome than the standard broiler breeds. It is common in America but some of the 'traditional free-range' birds (see page 87) on sale in the UK are of this breed.

GUINEA FOWL

Guinea fowl are members of the pheasant family, with a flavour somewhere between pheasant and chicken. This slightly gamy flavour comes from the bird's ability to graze, so that it gets much of its nutrition from grass, plants, worms and so on. Free-range guinea fowl has a much better flavour than broiler chicken but indoor birds are very little improvement, though they are considerably older than broilers when killed (63 to 70 days), giving them a slightly more mature taste.

TURKEY

Bronze turkey (Cambridge Bronze) is a more flavoursome, slow-growing breed than the basic white bird. The white meat is darker and firmer. The legs have black feathers which leave some black stubs after plucking, so sometimes they are referred to confusingly as 'black' turkeys. Unlike white turkey, bronze turkeys are still seasonal, generally available only around Christmas, and nearly always free-range.

Norfolk Black turkey has a similar flavour to bronze turkey and it also has black, stubbly legs. The breast is less plump than bronze turkey and it is less widely available.

DUCK

Aylesbury or Pekin are the standard duck breeds used in the UK. These mature quite quickly (in 49 days or so) and produce pale, quite fatty flesh.

Duckling are simply younger birds.

Barbary duck, also known as **Muscovy duck**, is a smaller, leaner breed with darker, gamier flesh, more like a wild duck (see page 145). They are slower to mature, reaching their slaughter weight between 70 and 84 days.

Mulard ducks are a new French-style crossbreed, meatier and leaner than the standard breeds. They are relatively slow-maturing ducks, slaughtered at around 90 days.

Gressingham and **Trelough ducks** are modern breeds which are smaller and more compact than the Aylesbury or Pekin and resemble the darker-fleshed, leaner French breeds in flavour.

'Second-feather' ducks are older birds that are not killed until they get their second feathers – between 84 and 90 days old. So they should have a fuller, more mature flavour. They are usually from free-range systems.

DIFFERENT GRADES OF FREE-RANGE BIRDS

'Free-range' is a widely abused term. Not all free-range birds are raised in the same way, so this category of poultry is full of nuances. Don't be fooled by birds described as **extensive indoor** or **barn reared**. Although this sneaks into the over-wide legal definition of free-range set by European regulations, these are effectively birds reared in broiler circumstances (described above) with just a few marginal improvements.

Other than that, there are three separate legal definitions of free-range. These apply to chicken, turkey, ducks, guinea fowl and geese. The amount of indoor and outdoor space allocated is different for each species of bird – turkeys are given more room than chickens and so on.

Plain old **free-range** means that birds, though kept in barns, must have daytime access to open-air runs covered in vegetation for at least half of their lives. They have more space to move around when inside than the standard table bird, and access through 'popholes' is defined in relation to the size of the shed – in other words the birds should be able to get out easily if they want. During the final fattening stage, 70 per cent of the birds' diet must be cereal. Feed is likely to be better quality than for the standard table bird (see page 80) but there is no legal restriction on the inclusion of animal proteins or growth-promoting medication. These birds are from fast-growing breeds that reach slaughter age rapidly.

This is a much more humane system than the one for standard table birds, but it is important to get the free-range element into proportion – half a life (28 days in the case of a chicken), some of which the bird *might* spend outdoors. There are still question marks over the quality of their diet. Breeds of chicken used in this type of free-range need to be fast growing, therefore they are modern breeds that are not renowned for flavour. Birds may still be kept in huge, industrial-sized flocks because there is no restriction on flock size. This makes it stressful for the birds because they cannot establish a natural pecking order, and it can also be hard for them to make the most of access to outdoors. The bulk of British free-range chicken is reared to this standard.

Traditional free-range birds have slightly less space indoors than basic free-range ones. This is because they have daytime access to twice the space outdoors from the age of at least six weeks. These birds have to come from breeds that are recognised to be slow growing and adapted to outdoor rearing, and they are considerably older than basic free-range birds when killed – in the case of turkey, for example, they are twice the age. There are restrictions both on the number of birds in the flock and the size of the shed, but these are still very large (4,800 chickens, 5,200 guinea fowl, 2,500 capons or turkeys).

This type of free-range bird comes from a more intrinsically flavoursome breed and takes longer to attain its end weight. The breed will also help the birds' ability to make the most of access to the natural feeding outdoors, where it will feel more at home than a modern, fast-growing breed. All that, added to the fact that it is much older at slaughter than the average broiler chicken, means that it should taste significantly better. Limits on size mean that these are smaller-scale operations where animal husbandry is likely to be better. Question marks still remain over diet, but since these are high-value birds which will sell for a premium price, most farmers will stick to a diet free from undesirable animal protein, though certain preventative medicines are very likely to be included. A small minority of supermarket free-range birds qualify for this category.

Free-range total freedom birds are just like traditional free-range except that they have continuous daytime access to open-air runs of unlimited area. A refinement on the above but likely to taste even better, since the birds will probably have better-quality vegetation on which to feed because it is more extensive. Their 'indoors' is more likely to be small henhouses which are moved over suitable land. This is the best system in animal welfare terms, and the closest to most consumers' image of free-range. Usually only imported (French) and small, local British producers' birds qualify for this category.

ORGANIC POULTRY

Organic birds have to conform to the strictest welfare standards. Flocks are much smaller in size (upper limit 500), which allows the birds to develop a natural pecking order, and encourages good husbandry. The birds must have continuous easy daytime access to outdoors. By its nature, organic poultry has to be free-range: indoor, intensive systems are out. All organic chickens, for example, will be kept in conditions that conform to either the 'traditional free-range' or 'free-range total freedom' requirements.

The diet of organic birds must be at least 70 per cent organic. The other 30 per cent can be made up of pulses and elements such as soya. (This is likely to be cut down as organic grain becomes more widely available.) Organic birds are often kept on traditional mixed farms which grow their own grain and where they can also feed on organic pastures. No animal protein is permitted.

All routine veterinary medicines are prohibited except for the brief use, for young chicks, of a medicine to control coccidiosis (a common infection in birds), which would otherwise affect their growth. Long, slow growth means that chickens, for example, will take around 90 days to reach their ideal slaughter weight.

A high-quality diet, combined with a free-ranging lifestyle from a very early age, makes organic poultry some of the best-tasting you can expect to find. Since the word 'organic' is often bandied about indiscriminately, only buy birds from producers certified by the Soil Association or another recognised certifying body (see page 284).

THE GOOSE: MORE SMART THAN SILLY

The goose is the one species of farmed poultry that has mounted a resistance to factory farming. They are strongly protective, easily frightened, need warmth, and become ill readily if not well-treated, so they are complicated birds to rear. This means they cannot be raised intensively and so all geese are effectively outdoors birds, kept in largely natural circumstances. Left to peck away at good pasture, they can feed themselves on grass alone. Most goose producers, however, do feed them cereals, vitamins and minerals.

It is doubtless within the bounds of possibility that

some bright-spark animal breeder could devise a means of rearing the difficult goose intensively. Fortunately, there is little commercial drive to do so, since the relatively small amount of meat and large amount of fat on a goose make it of limited appeal to consumers accustomed to poultry bred for huge amounts of cheap, lean breast meat.

So the small number of geese reared in the UK remain naturally free-range birds. This makes them a flavoursome, seasonal treat for the discerning consumer. Geese are strictly seasonal, available first for Michaelmas (end of September), with progressively more plump birds through to Christmas.

TRACKING DOWN A BETTER TURKEY

Turkey used to be strictly a Christmas bird but the growth of intensive turkey farming has put paid to all that, with standard white turkeys now on sale throughout the year. However, Christmas still remains the best time for really good turkeys. Free-range and organic producers, farmers who concentrate on the more flavoursome breeds like the Bronze and Norfolk Black, still gear their production to Christmas.

One better kind of Christmas turkey if you cannot find organic or free-range is **Gold Triangle Turkey**, which comes with a consumer guarantee from the Traditional Farmfresh Turkey Association, an alliance of independent farmers. The Gold Triangle goes on birds that have been kept in better circumstances. Some, though not all, are free-range, so there are two different types of gold triangle logo.

Indoor birds qualifying for this triangle have to be kept in buildings with both natural light and ventilation, regularly bedded with straw and wood shavings and slaughtered on the farm to avoid distress from long-distance transport. Though their initial diet may contain fish meal, they eat at least 70 per cent cereals thereafter. These birds do receive routine medicine in their feed to combat common diseases but the emphasis is on keeping these to a minimum.

Unlike the majority of Christmas turkeys, these birds are dry-plucked (hand-plucked), resulting in a good smooth skin, and are hung up to mature for 7 to 21 days. This means that, like meat, they develop a better flavour and become more tender. Most turkeys are wet-plucked (by machine), then sold without maturing.

POULTRY AND THE RISK OF FOOD POISONING

Two food-poisoning bacteria are endemic in poultry: salmonella and campylobacter. They flourish when birds are farmed intensively and are hard to eliminate.

The bugs can cause anything from a mild stomach upset to death – though this is very rare – depending on the degree of contamination and the victim's state of health. Tests frequently show that a significant percentage of birds are contaminated. Salmonella has been found in over a third of samples and campylobacter in around 40 per cent. It is thought that only two out of every five chickens, for example, can be given the all-clear for both bacteria.

When buying poultry, obviously you cannot see if it is infected, but you can reduce the risk of food poisoning.

- Buy traditional free-range or organic poultry. Birds kept in more extensive circumstances are less likely to be contaminated, partly because they are less crammed together but also because they are older at slaughter, so their immune systems are more able to fight bacteria.

- Avoid cheap poultry products made from re-formed scraps (see below). These carry a higher risk of contamination.
- Buy poultry very fresh and cook it straight away. Do not leave it hanging around in your fridge.
- Make sure the bird is thoroughly cooked. The juices should run clear if you insert a knife near the thigh bone.
- If using frozen poultry, make sure that it is completely defrosted before cooking.
- Do not let poultry drip on to other food in the fridge. Wash chopping utensils and work surfaces well after contact.
- Be wary of microwave ovens. Many models have 'cold spots', which means that food-poisoning bugs are not killed off as they are in conventional ovens.
- Do not partly cook and then reheat chicken.

POULTRY BURGERS, SAUSAGES AND RE-FORMED MEAT PRODUCTS

Chicken and turkey meat have been one of the commercial success stories of the last decade, because they are lean, cheap and versatile. These characteristics have been harnessed in a whole range of 'added-value' products – burgers, nuggets, drummers, kievs, sausages, rolls and joints. And yet these items are extremely low quality.

For starters, the turkey and chicken used in these products is always from the most intensively kept birds (see page 80). Then there is the type of poultry 'meat' used. First there is **re-formed meat**, which is bits of white or brown meat that have been chopped up, massaged, tumbled and bound together with a variety of additives so that they hold together in a pre-ordained shape. That is superior to **mechanically recovered meat (MRM)**. This is a sort of poultry slurry obtained by subjecting the carcass (after normal butchery) to such hydraulic or centrifugal pressure that the residue meat texture is changed to allow it to flow off the bone. It is sometimes also known as mechanically separated meat.

Once all the regular meat has been removed, the carcasses still retain small scraps of meat, sinew and connective tissue. Obtained in this way it is a fairly revolting substance, but mixed in with re-formed meat, breadcrumbed, battered and 'seasoned' with flavour-enhancing additives, it can bulk out products and make a tidy profit for manufacturers. Most manufacturers now declare MRM on the label, although there is, as yet, no legal obligation to do so.

These types of poultry products are low-grade food and, though cheap, usually represent bad value for money. They are risky from the food poisoning point of view, too, because any sort of chopping or mincing process breaks down the chemical stability of meat and instantly makes it more susceptible to harmful bacteria. Both salmonella and campylobacter are frequently present in the cheap, intensive poultry used to make these products, so these processes heighten the risk. MRM is especially dodgy, since meat around the carcass is known to contain more harmful bacteria than other bits.

Many products containing MRM are sold as 'cook from frozen'. This can aggravate the risk even further because it is harder to cook the meat right through and kill off the bacteria. This is especially the case with microwaves.

FROZEN POULTRY

Watch out for water...

Most poultry is 'wet-plucked' which means that it is done by machine, not by hand. Since quite a lot of water is needed to wash, pluck and then chill a bird, some of that is absorbed into the carcass. If the bird is then frozen, even more water is absorbed, which adversely affects the taste.

There are regulations covering the water content of frozen chickens but none for turkeys or other poultry, so many a frozen bird is waterlogged by the time you get it. It is best to buy poultry fresh but if you have to buy it frozen, try to find a bird that is 'air chill' or 'air-spray chill' frozen rather than 'immersion' frozen – literally frozen in water.

This information does not have to be declared on the label but some more upmarket brands will indicate the type of freezing. Price is a guide too; immersion-frozen birds are the cheapest around.

Be aware of the age...

The average frozen turkey will have been frozen for about two years by the time you buy it, some may have been stored frozen for as long as five years. Shocked? It's perfectly legal because there is no legal 'best-before' limit for frozen turkeys. A freezing date would be helpful to the consumer but there is little chance of this happening.

There is no evidence that turkey deteriorates during years of freezing, but it is just another reason for favouring fresh.

Eggs

Few of our core foodstuffs have been more compromised than the egg. Finding the proverbial 'good egg' produced by a hen in anything approaching natural circumstances is like looking for a needle in a haystack. Humane systems of egg production – ones that treat the hen with respect, not as a production-line component which can be disposed of when worn out – are few and far between. The harsh reality of egg production in Britain today is that the vast majority of our eggs come from miserable, much-abused birds, kept in squalid circumstances where disease is often endemic.

Unfortunately, not enough consumers are aware of this, or egg producers would have a revolution on their hands and standards would inevitably be improved. Most of us trustingly buy those vaguely comforting 'farm-fresh', 'country', 'breakfast' assurances that we see on the typical egg box next to idyllic, fairy-tale images of sunny farmyards with contented hens and chicks. These are not regulated by law and are meaningless. Only a minority of eggs name the farm they come from, and although that might give a more rustic impression you cannot automatically assume that they are any better than those that do not. The Co-op has developed a much more candid label for battery eggs – 'intensively produced' – and there is pressure for other retailers to follow suit. Meanwhile, the almost total absence of any concrete information on labels explaining when and how eggs have been produced makes it extremely difficult to differentiate between various sorts.

How most eggs are produced – the battery cage

About 88 per cent of the eggs on sale in the UK are produced in a battery cage. Unless the box says 'free-range', 'barn' or 'organic', you can assume that you are buying battery eggs. This is a completely inhumane system whose only 'virtue' is that it provides cheap eggs. It is widely discredited both in the UK and internationally and should be scrapped.

Battery houses are large, windowless sheds which offer inadequate fresh air and no daylight. Each one houses anything from 30,000 to over 100,000 birds. The hens are kept in a series of wire cages which are arranged in rows and stacked on top of each other. They are crowded four or five to a cage measuring 43 by 48 centimetres. They cannot spread their wings out or turn around freely. Needless to say, flying is totally impossible.

Hens have very strong instincts to scratch the ground, to dust-bathe, to perch, to make nests and to preen themselves. All these needs are frustrated in the battery cage. Battery hens stand on wire for 24 hours each day. (Wire is needed to let the droppings fall through, but it also damages the eggs.) The hens have no exercise, so many suffer from brittle bones, making them susceptible to injury. Claw and leg deformities are common because the hen is standing on wire, day in, day out.

Because the hens are unable to satisfy their basic instincts in this barren environment they become bored and aggressive. They start pecking each other – a symptom of frustration which can escalate into cannibalism. In order to prevent this, battery houses are permanently lit. But this is not usually enough, so the hens often have part of their beaks cut off with a red-hot blade. The egg industry attempts to justify the battery cage on the grounds that it cuts down the need for de-beaking. But independent sources say that this mutilation is nevertheless routinely carried out on all one-day-old chicks. It is known to cause chronic long-term pain and suffering for the birds. The hens live in these appalling circumstances for about a year, where there are many casualties and deaths.

In a year the typical hen produces up to 300 eggs, at which point she will be 'spent' – so clapped-out that her meat is only fit for low-grade food processing uses (cat food, spreads, stock cubes, tinned soup and so on).

WHAT BATTERY HENS EAT: 'FOOD', MEDICINES AND COLOURINGS

In the natural order of things, hens would peck around in grass or woodland and this diet would be supplemented with wholesome grain by the farmer. Battery hens never go outdoors and are fed instead on 'rations' containing grain (mainly wheat and barley), soya, vitamins, minerals and a few other unsavoury extras. These can legally include meat and bone meal derived from the carcasses of dead animals, fish meal, feather meal and blood meal from poultry slaughterhouses.

This compromised diet and the unnatural circumstances of intensive production mean that hens are not as healthy as they should be and are therefore more vulnerable to disease. So rations are routinely medicated to prevent outbreaks of illness. Poultry farmers and feed merchants are extremely reticent about revealing the contents of the feed, but medicines used include antibiotics, coccidiostats and aspirin. Synthetic amino acids are also added for extra protein to encourage better rates of production.

In classic farmyard circumstances, hens produce eggs with yolks all different shades of yellow, depending on the season and what they have been eating. In the battery system, yolks are all the same consistent colour, since yellow colourings are added to the feed according to the wholesaler's preference. Some of the colours are naturally derived – from marigold petals and paprika, for example – although these would not normally be found in eggs. Artificial colours used in poultry feed have question marks over their toxicity. Either way, the presence of these colourings does not have to be declared on the label.

Non-battery eggs: the better 12 per cent?

What about the remaining 12 per cent or thereabouts of eggs which are not produced in batteries? In this category, it is even harder for consumers to know what they are getting. In theory, these are the better eggs, produced with some basic commitment to animal welfare and the concept of producing wholesome, nourishing food. However, there are many different standards operating, ranging from very minor reforms of the battery system which may, in total, be just as bad for the birds, to others that are genuinely enlightened. Since most eggs are not labelled with the farm or even the country they have come from, let alone details of the production methods, it is almost impossible for the consumer to tell them apart. Most of the terms used sound a lot better than the reality. As a general rule, read the label carefully and buy eggs that give you the maximum amount of information indicating welfare awareness, content of feed and so on.

BARN EGGS

Barn eggs have become the industry's answer to consumer criticisms of battery cages. Like battery hens, barn hens spend their entire time indoors. Some barns have windows to allow in a certain amount of daylight, but many are just renovated battery houses where the cages have been dismantled and replaced with wooden perches and, in some systems, nesting boxes. In theory, the birds are freer to move around, fly, and use the space available to them. It should mean that they are also less prone to claw and leg injuries, since they are not standing permanently on thin wire.

The problem with most barn systems, however, is that they are often stocked with as many hens as battery houses. This means that the hens are still severely overcrowded, and kept in flocks that are far too large. Barn systems are therefore particularly likely to cause cannibalism, feather-pecking and aggression, with weaker hens having even less protection than in the battery cage. Hens in barn systems may eat each other's droppings and their own eggs, and frequently lay their eggs on the floor instead of in the nesting boxes.

In all other ways, barn hens are subject to the same indignities as battery hens. De-beaking is routine, and there is no reason to suppose that their diet is any better. All in all, barn eggs (which represent a measly 3–4 per cent of British egg production), though preferable to battery eggs, are no great step forward in terms of either bird welfare or egg quality.

FREE-RANGE EGGS – A MINIMUM GUARANTEE

While most consumers fondly think of free-range as a spacious, overwhelmingly outdoor system, the reality is often far from that. For a system to qualify as free-range, hens must be given continuous notional access to outdoors. Unfortunately that is often where the liberty ends.

The European Union standards for free-range eggs are pathetically low. Hens can be kept in their thousands in huge, industrial-sized flocks and stocked even more densely than battery hens. The legal minimum affords each 'free-range' hen an area of 29 by 19 centimetres. This is because these regulations are based on the space traditionally given to genuinely free-range birds who spend most of the day outdoors, using the henhouse only at night. (When hens are outside for most of the time, much less indoor space is required.) Modern breeds of egg-laying hen are often not able to make the most of the access to outdoors. They have been bred to be more passive and they are stocked so densely, in such huge industrial sheds, that their natural instinct to go outside is frustrated. So they often end up staying inside.

In certain systems, the access to outdoors is through a series of narrow 'popholes', with more dominant hens clustered all around, so many hens are scared to go out. If they do venture outside, there is no guarantee that the land is suitable. It should be covered in vegetation: grass, natural woodland and so on. Many pseudo free-range birds only get out on to the factory-farm equivalent of a building site – concrete, asphalt and so on. Are free-range eggs better in other respects? They might be, but you cannot take that for granted. Free-range hens usually have their beaks cut too. This obviously inhibits them from pecking up food from outdoors and making the most of their free-range potential.

Apart from a glimpse of outdoors, they may be given nothing in an otherwise barren environment to help them fulfil their natural instincts. There is no legal obligation to provide nests, perches or litter to scratch in, although in practice, these are generally provided. Free-range hens usually eat the same unsavoury diet as their battery and barn equivalents, too.

HOW TO SPOT BETTER FREE-RANGE SYSTEMS

The best eggs are likely to come from the few good free-range systems. The hallmarks of these are the opposite of the systems described above. The hens should spend most of their time outside on suitable land, only returning to henhouses at night. They should be fed a natural and nutritious diet, free from recycled animal protein waste, drugs and colourings.

Relatively few British producers offer eggs to this standard. Those who do generally label them with a quality guarantee which gives many more details about production methods, a more specific idea of the land and area over which the hens roam, and assurances about the content of their feed. Good free-range eggs like these are generally found in small specialist or wholefood shops, often accompanied by explanatory leaflets and posters.

ORGANIC EGGS

Organic eggs are currently very few and far between but if you can track them down they are a good bet. Beak clipping is banned and battery and barn systems are not permitted. Hens must be given generous indoor space and have easy, continuous access to outdoors. To prevent stress, the maximum permitted flock size is 500. The pasture on which the hens feed must be rested one year out of every three to prevent the build up of parasites. At least 70 per cent of the birds' diet must be organically produced, while other feed must be from permitted natural sources. Preventative antibiotics, animal proteins and wastes and yolk colourants are banned.

Organic eggs should all carry a symbol or stamp showing that they are approved by an organic certifying body (see page 284). Watch out for frauds. It is easy to put a few eggs in a rustic-looking basket and call them 'organic' just because they are better in one minor respect. Even eggs from organic farms may not be strictly organic, because the organic approval may extend only to other produce, such as vegetables. Only buy eggs that have a clear organic certification.

'VEGETARIAN' EGGS

A small number of eggs are sold with a 'V' symbol, indicating that they have been approved by the Vegetarian Society. These eggs come with a guarantee that the hens have been fed on natural foodstuffs, with no medicines, colourings or animal protein. In addition, they must fulfil quite demanding free-range requirements. They are available in specialist and wholefood shops.

FOUR-GRAIN EGGS

These eggs come with a guarantee that the hens have been fed only on natural foodstuffs with no animal protein. Although the feed contains colourings, no medicines are included. This is a useful assurance to have but it does not mean you can assume the eggs are free-range. Although the hens have had a much healthier and more nutritious diet, they are still kept in the barn system. Most upmarket supermarket branches stock four-grain eggs.

'FREEDOM FOOD' EGGS

These eggs are sold with a guarantee from the RSPCA that the hens have been free from:

- hunger and thirst
- discomfort
- pain, injury and disease
- fear and distress.

In addition, the hens must have freedom to express normal behaviour.

Though an improvement on the worst excesses of intensive egg production, in practice these conditions are very weak. For example, although a hen may not be actively hungry or thirsty, she may still be receiving an unbalanced diet.

Eggs bearing this logo cannot come from a battery cage system but they may still come from barn and perchery systems (see page 99), which are extremely intensive and where the hens never go outdoors. Beak-clipping is still permitted. Animal protein in feed is banned but this may lead to even greater use of synthetic amino acids, which are not properly part of a hen's natural diet but are used to produce even bigger eggs. Yolk colourings and antibiotics may still be included, too. Certain supermarket chains stock Freedom Food eggs.

HENS' EGGS WITH DIFFERENT SHELLS

Some supermarkets now sell **'Speckledy hens' eggs'**. These shiny, brown-shelled eggs come from hens that have been crossed with older, more traditional breeds. Some people think that they have a better taste than the average hen's egg, and because the hens are less productive than modern breeds the eggs cost more.

Eggs like these appeal to the consumer who wants a more 'natural' egg. As a rule, they have been produced by hens fed on an improved diet (like the four-grain egg) but, unless it states explicitly on the box, they are unlikely to be free-range and will normally be barn eggs. Upmarket supermarket branches stock them.

White eggs are rarely seen these days because there is a British preference for brown ones. White eggs come from different breeds of chicken than brown ones. At one time, industrial eggs were all white and so brown eggs come to be associated with farmyard, free-range eggs and were seen as superior. Nowadays most egg producers – be they intensive, free-range or organic – produce only brown eggs. White and brown eggs are exactly the same nutritionally.

DOUBLE-YOLKED EGGS

Double-yolked eggs occur when a hen produces two yolks from her ovaries at the same time. These are therefore larger than normal eggs, the ratio of white to yolk is not as it should be, and the shell will be thinner, more porous, and therefore more prone to contamination. These eggs have not developed as they should and are therefore considered an abnormality.

Double-yolked eggs used to be selected out as second-quality eggs and sold for baking or other uses. They were relatively rare. These days hens have been made more productive by being given high-protein feed and kept in battery sheds with bright lighting. This encourages them into early laying and results in more eggs. They are bred increasingly to produce bigger eggs, too, which means that many more hens may be producing double-yolked eggs than before.

Far from being graded as second quality, double-yolked eggs are now commonly sold in boxes of six, as if they were something special – probably because there are too many of them to sell as second grade. In a smart box or not, the same objections still stand.

QUAIL, DUCK AND GOOSE EGGS

Don't assume that quail's eggs are any better or more natural than hen's eggs. Despite their attractive speckled appearance, almost all of them are produced in every bit as intensive and unsavoury circumstances as hen's eggs. Duck and goose eggs are not produced commercially, so if you can find them there is a high chance that they will have come from a small-scale farm and been laid by free-ranging birds.

RAW EGG RISKS

Salmonella is endemic in chickens and therefore common in eggs. This is widely regarded as a consequence of the squalid, unhealthy conditions in which most hens are kept. Eggs (and chicken) are the commonest source of food poisoning in the UK. As a result, you court danger each time you eat a raw or lightly cooked egg, since the bacteria will not have been killed off by cooking. To be absolutely safe, you need to cook eggs until the yolk is firm.

For this reason, it is extremely unwise to eat raw or lightly cooked eggs if you are old, pregnant or have reduced immunity to disease through illness. Some authorities go as far as recommending that people eliminate raw eggs from their diet altogether. Many catering operations have replaced raw egg with pasteurised dried egg to ensure safety. Unfortunately, these substitutes taste horrible by comparison.

Since raw eggs are essential for a number of dishes – mayonnaise, cold mousses, eggnogs and so on – it is hard to eliminate them entirely. And if you are in good health, you may be prepared to take the risk.

If you eat raw or lightly cooked eggs, make sure that they are as fresh as possible and have been kept cool. A cold, moist, old-fashioned larder is the ideal store. Failing this, keep them at the top of your refrigerator or in the door. Refrigerated eggs should be left at room temperature for 30 minutes before cooking.

Salmonella in eggs multiplies quickly with age. Very fresh eggs – even if they are contaminated – will contain lower levels of bacteria and are more likely to make you only slightly, rather than severely, ill. Never use eggs raw if you have had them for more than five days. Always discard eggs with any cracks or slight signs of shell damage. Dirty eggs are a sign of a bad production system; don't buy them. Check the provenance of your eggs, too, and try to buy genuine free-range eggs, which are less likely to be contaminated in the first place.

JUDGING THE FRESHNESS OF EGGS

All eggs are sold with a **'best before' date**. This is actually quite dangerous, particularly for people who still eat raw eggs, because is does not tell you the **laying date**. Some retailers now put the **packing date** on eggs, which consumers often mistake for the laying date. In theory, the 'best before' date should be calculated on the basis of 21 days after the packing date which should be the same or, at worst, the next day after laying day. So if you wanted to check the exact age of your eggs, you should be able to subtract 21 days from the 'best before' date, then add on the number of days between that and today. In practice, however, the packing date can be anything up to 10 days *after* laying. Packing stations are not obliged to pick up eggs from farms more than once a week and they can sit at the packing station for a further three days. There is no legal limit on the 'best before' date. Some egg companies use 28 days from laying, not 21 days. Add a 10-day lapse between packing and laying and it is perfectly possible for your eggs to be four to six weeks old before you buy them!

The absence of a legally required laying date makes it impossible for consumers to judge the freshness of eggs, and this is essential information. While a nearly three-week-old egg might be just about acceptable for baking in a cake, for example, it is simply not fresh enough for lightly scrambled or runny eggs and absolutely out of the question for eating raw.

Some retailers sell **'superfresh'** and **'extra fresh'** eggs. These are guaranteed to have been laid and packed on the same day – not much more than one might expect anyway! More importantly, they are sent to stores within a couple of days and taken off the shelves sooner if they haven't sold. Such eggs are definitely fresher than most but that does not give you any further guarantee about how the hen was kept, what she ate and so on.

A GOOD FRESH EGG

Crack open a really fresh egg and the yolk should plop out, then rest high, proud and intact on top of the white. The white should be thick, jelly-like and hold its shape as well as supporting the yolk. If the egg pours out of the shell, the yolk breaks on contact with the bowl and the white is runny and watery, it is not fresh. Very old eggs will float if you put them in a bowl of water, while fresher ones will sit on the bottom. However, this is a very basic test and should only be used to weed out eggs that are not fit for use of any sort, not as a guarantee of freshness.

THE SIZE OF EGGS

Though eggs are sold by size, size is really measured by weight. Every egg must be weighed, then put into one of seven different bands, each of which is only 5 grams different. Though you might see a difference between the smallest egg and the largest one, the difference between a size-3 and a size-4 egg is negligible. Using one size rather than another will not make any perceptible impact on your recipe.

Meat

The pedigree of most meat on sale in the UK is a bit of a mystery. Apart from the country of origin, you'll be lucky to get any hard information. Many retailers themselves are ignorant of the provenance of their meat, simply buying from the abattoir in the form of anonymous carcasses or ready-to-cut sections.

When we buy meat like this we tend to assume optimistically that it will be of good average quality. These 'silent' labels appeal to a safety-in-numbers philosophy. We like to think that behind them lie lots of reassuring points, which the packers just forgot to tell us.

If this was ever the case, it certainly isn't now. The odd insights we get into the secretive standards behind those 'oven-ready turkeys', 'prime pork' and so on suggest that we should be distrustful. Anyone who is producing the best or simply better quality meat these days – and there are more every day – is letting us know about it. Good meat comes with a pedigree and a history. Labels are becoming more informative, while accompanying leaflets and propaganda try to answer our concerns – animal welfare, food safety, eating quality and so on.

Good meat is the end product of a patient, careful process. The animal should come from a traditional breed that is known for its eating quality. Such animals flourish best in outdoor systems where they can exercise properly, taking advantage of fresh air, daylight and natural feeding. They should reach their end weight slowly. When slaughtered, they should be transported and killed in such a way that they suffer no stress – the meat will be affected otherwise. Then the meat needs to be hung, or matured, so that it eats well.

Bad meat is the unsatisfactory product of a fast-track farming system which rewards output rather than quality. It favours breeds of animals that have been developed to be extremely productive and to have what farmers call a high 'feed conversion' rate – at the expense of flavour. This type of production is just one big rush to the slaughterhouse. The animals have to put on weight quickly, something that is encouraged by the feeding of high-protein foods and routine medication which would not naturally be part of their diets. It is easiest to control this indoors, so the animals cannot exercise properly or take advantage of fresh air and daylight. Having reached optimum weight in record time, it's off to the slaughterhouse or the market, without any great concern about stress or suffering entailed. Once on the hook, time is money and the luxury of maturing the meat is simply not justified.

It is becoming ever more obvious that the welfare of the animal and the end quality of the meat are two sides of the same coin. They are influenced by a number of factors:
- the breed of the animal
- what it has eaten
- whether it has been raised indoors or outdoors
- its ability to exercise (predicated on the above)
- the way it has been transported and slaughtered
- the manner in which the meat has been matured post-slaughter. So buy meat with a label that specifies the maximum amount of information on these important issues.

A WORD ABOUT OFFAL...

Liver, kidney, sweetbreads, tongue, brain, etc. – some love them, some hate them. Whatever your preference, and whatever the animal, it is worth remembering that these products are more likely to harbour traces of both legal and illegal drugs. Europe-wide studies show that we have at least three times more chance of eating residues of illegal drugs (growth promoters, antibiotics, etc.) in offal such as liver than in muscle meat such as steak. Some cattle offals are no longer on sale because of worries that they might harbour the infectious agent responsible for BSE (mad cow disease).

If you enjoy eating offal, be very sure of your source.

Beef

Is beef wholesome food, or is it mad, bad and potentially dangerous? The problem for the consumer is that 'beef' is a very broad category. It includes some of the most delicious, naturally reared meat around but also some of the worst excesses of intensive farming, produced at the expense of animal welfare, food quality and possibly human health.

THE BEST BEEF

The best-quality beef is from herds of cattle reared specifically for this purpose, from breeds that are only used for beef, not milk (see page 113). Farmers call them 'beef-suckler herds'. They are reared in a traditional way, which means that they spend their summers outside, grazing on good pasture, the calves kept with their mothers and drinking their milk until they are old enough to graze for themselves. In winter they may remain outside, although some are brought into warm, protected barns with a good bedding of clean straw and fed on high-quality food – silage (preserved grass), vegetables, grains and added vitamins and minerals. Most beef cattle are killed at between 18 months and two years, having spent a lot of their lives outdoors eating a very natural diet. Older cattle, kept for breeding purposes, often live to eight years old or more. Ultimately, beef-suckler animals sell for a substantial sum of money, so it is in the farmer's interest to see that they are well cared for. They are usually slaughtered more humanely, too, since poor slaughter results in tough meat because of stress to the animal – this would undo all the farmers' good work and the meat would not achieve a premium price.

This is the traditional way of rearing beef throughout Scotland. The quality of animal husbandry is high and the meat quality can be glorious, hence the worldwide reputation of Scotch beef.

A little beef is produced from suckler herds in other parts of the UK but it is a much smaller proportion of all beef. Although beef from suckler herds makes up 68 per cent of Scottish beef production, it makes up only 25 per cent of English, and 40 per cent of UK beef production.

However, this kind of beef is becoming more popular with farmers throughout the UK as consumers raise more questions about the quality of meat they are buying. Any good butcher should be able to tell you whether his or her beef is from beef-suckler herds. The best can even name the farm from which it came. Another guide is price. Traditional beef costs more, but the taste should be much better. Supermarkets have developed a number of different labels, including 'speciality', 'heritage', 'traditional' and so on to delineate a superior type of beef. Such labels usually go some, but not all the way to meet the demands of the welfare-/quality-minded consumer. The supermarkets make them up and they have no legal or independent definition, although most are an improvement on unspecified 'beef'. Read the label carefully. The selling points will be prominent but they may leave other questions unanswered. Measure your label against the list of factors influencing the quality of meat on page 109. It will probably match up on certain grounds and be silent on others. Use these labels as indicators of improvements, but don't automatically assume they offer a total guarantee.

ORGANIC BEEF

Organic beef is a refinement on the traditional product of the beef herds described above, the main difference being that the calves must feed on pasture that has not been treated with chemicals. This means that organic calves graze some of the finest and most natural pasture around. If brought indoors, they are fed in the same way as traditional beef herds but this too must be at least 90 per cent organic. At least 60 per cent of the dry matter has to come from forage, which means that intensive barley-beef systems (see page 114) are not permitted. Animal welfare standards are strict and give more protection to calves, particularly in the vexed area of live transport between farms. Winter housing has to be provided for the cattle in areas where weather conditions can be severe. Routine drugs and antibiotic growth promoters are not allowed.

If you can get it – usually direct from the farmer – organic beef is likely to be excellent. Make sure it is has an organic guarantee (see page 284). Some supermarkets stock organic beef, clearly labelled as such.

JUDGING THE QUALITY OF BEEF

To eat well, beef needs to be hung for anything from 14 to 21 days, depending on how tender you like it. Good beef should be purplish-red, quite dark as it matures, and the lean meat should have a nice marbling of fat through it. The fat should be creamy-white, though in grass-fed beef it may be more yellow in appearance. The more it matures, the firmer and dryer the meat will become. Beef that is bright red and moist looking is probably young and has not been hung for long. Some butchers prefer to sell meat this way. Beef loses weight as it dries out, and so the butcher can see lengthy hanging as a loss-making exercise.

The Meat and Livestock Commission recommends that butchers hang their meat for seven to ten days, and this is now standard supermarket and high-street practice.

Many top butchers think beef should be hung for 14 to 21 days to develop a more pronounced taste and reliable tenderness. They usually charge a little more to compensate for any weight loss. Ask your butcher what his or her policy is.

Increasingly, supermarkets are selling joints or cuts of beef in transparent pre-packs filled with nitrogen and carbon dioxide gas. This prevents the oxygen naturally present in air from darkening the meat, so it won't look like the traditional beef described above. 'Gas flushing' of meat does not need to be declared on the label, and will certainly slow down the normal development of a piece of beef, giving it a much longer shelf life. Usually supermarkets using this technique have matured the meat first by sophisticated hanging and chilling methods. It may be tender, even though it looks too young – eating it is the only test!

THE BEST-TASTING BREEDS

The finest beef comes from traditional, dedicated beef breeds, the most outstanding of which is the legendary **Aberdeen Angus**. It is thought that the 'black Angus', as it is sometimes known, carries a gene which produces fine threads of creamy white fat interwoven through the red meat, making it succulent and tender when cooked. **Highland** and **Beef Shorthorn** offer close competition. **Hereford, Galloway** and the red breeds (**Devon, Lincoln** and **Sussex reds**) all produce beef of some distinction. Like the Aberdeen Angus, these breeds are fatter than the 'modern' ones introduced from the Continent, which produce leaner, but less flavoursome meat.

DAIRY BEEF – WELL WORTH AVOIDING

Two kinds of beef are undesirable in terms of both food quality and animal welfare because they come from the same basic source – dairy animals. This meat is a by-product of the dairy industry and is quite different from the traditional beef-suckler herds described above, because:

- The breeds used (mainly Friesians and Holstein) are chosen for the large quantities of milk they produce, not their meat.
- They are generally intensively farmed compared to suckler herds.

   Meat from these sources benefits from neither the breeding, feeding, nor outdoor life associated with good beef. About 60 per cent of the beef sold in the UK is a by-product of dairy herds and you can assume that this is what you are buying unless it is labelled as beef from beef herds.

Barley beef

The first type of beef derived from dairy herds is what is known as barley beef. Dairy calves are separated from their mothers soon after birth and fed on a substitute liquid diet until they are old enough to be given cereals and protein supplements. This type of feeding is not natural and can often result in metabolic diseases and liver damage. All this production goes on indoors in tightly packed sheds. If the calves are lucky they may be given some straw, but many spend most of their lives on concrete or slatted floors. By this means, calves can reach their optimum weight at around 12 months, thus giving the farmer a better return on investment. Some production of this kind is less intensive than others. Farmers may put the calves out to grass for a few weeks or so but their lives are still substantially more restricted than beef-suckler equivalents. Calves raised in this way are often moved around a lot, passing through live animal markets and different rearing and finishing (fattening) units. There is evidence to suggest that in the process, such calves are not always well treated.

Apart from objections on animal welfare grounds, the diet of these calves is of particular concern to consumers. The grass the calves would normally eat is replaced by barley and they are also fed on high-protein concentrates, designed to boost production levels. These can legally contain a number of undesirable extras, such as dried skimmed milk powder, dried blood flavoured with chocolate, fish meal (ground-up fish) and dried poultry manure (DPM), which consists of used chicken litter, feather waste and dead carcasses of intensive poultry that have been recycled.

Since meat and bone meal from animal sources is thought to be a likely cause of mad cow disease (see page 119), it is no longer legal to feed cows protein or recycled waste from sheep, pigs or other cattle. However, animal protein from poultry sources is still permitted. The government has also admitted that some banned feedstuffs have been used illegally by farmers.

A range of **antibiotic growth promoters** is routinely used in barley-beef production and there is concern that these might provoke immunity in humans to certain groups of antibiotics commonly used for human health.

The use of **growth-promoting hormones** has been banned in Europe but there is widespread evidence that illegal beta-agonist drugs, such as clenbuterol ('angel dust') are being used by unscrupulous farmers as a profitable shortcut to production. Residues turn up with frightening regularity in beef, especially in liver.

Old dairy cow beef

Dairy cows are deemed to have come to the end of their prematurely short lives at around six to seven years, as opposed to a natural lifespan of 20 or more, because their milk yield has dropped. By this stage, as well as being economically unproductive, the cows are worn out through being kept in an unnatural state of continuous lactation and pregnancy (see Milk and Dairy Products). These cows are then 'culled' (slaughtered) and their tough old meat is still considered by the powers that be as fit to eat.

If you were eating a chicken you would doubtless prefer to select one that had been raised for the table, not a spent egg-laying hen. Old cow beef is the beef equivalent. At very best, the meat from tired-out milkers is bound to be tough. But old dairy cows will also have eaten more of the less desirable animal feed-stuffs described above, which are implicated as possible sources of BSE (mad cow disease). In addition, throughout their lives they will have been given routine medication in their feed to keep them productive. This means that their meat is the lowest quality around and possibly hazardous.

Old cow beef is not labelled in any way that the consumer can recognise but it usually goes to one of two outlets – catering, including canteens and school meals, and food processing (see below).

One other product – **gelatine** – is derived from the skin and bones of old cows. It is of an extremely dubious nature and best avoided (see page 236).

MINCE AND CHEAPER BEEF PRODUCTS

As a rule of thumb, if you want good-quality beef, products such as mince, sausages, burgers, faggots, bridies, meat pies and pasties are least likely to offer it. Obviously there are exceptions. Butchers buying the best traditional beef from beef-suckler herds have to use up the scraps of the meat that the consumer doesn't buy – and very tasty they can be too. It is only common sense, after all, to avoid waste by transforming it into a sausage or some other eco-nomical product.

However, the minute meat is processed out of its original state, it opens the door for food adulteration. It is not always easy to tell the good from the bad.

Whether you are buying mince, burgers, faggots or sausages from an independent butcher, supermarket or freezer shop, the question you should always ask is, what is the quality of the basic meat? **Minced beef**, or **mince**, should legally be made from 100 per cent minced beef with no more than 25 per cent added beef fat. (Steak mince should be 100 per cent from cuts that you could eat as a steak.) **Beef products** such as burgers and sausages are covered by a legal 'minimum meat declaration' and should be at least 80 per cent meat, although a proportion of that can be other meat (usually pork) unless it says 'all-beef'.

However, when mince is labelled as 100 per cent beef, or a beef product as 80 per cent beef, do not make the mistake of thinking that this is from prime cuts. Meat in both fresh mince and beef products can come from several sources, depending on the product. These include meat scraps from trimmed carcasses and parts of the animal most consumers don't want, such as tail meat, head meat, cheek, neck, shin, tongue, kidney, gristle and sinew. The UK permits looser standards than most other European countries when it comes to mince. It allows many more parts of the animal to be included in the composition of beef mince on the basis that our mince is bought to be cooked, while on the Continent beef may be eaten raw. This is why British mince contains more connective tissue and collagen than Continental mince. Eaten raw, this would be too chewy but when cooked it breaks down into gelatine.

Mince and beef products can also be made from old dairy cow beef, 'beef mountain' beef that has been frozen in intervention stocks for a number of years and then sold off cheaply, frozen imported beef and mechanically recovered or mechanically separated beef (MRM) – a meat slurry (see page 93). It is not thought that MRM is widely used in mince bought from butcher's shops, though, since it is sold in very large quantities and mainly bought by large processors.

MRM is under review by the European Commission and may at some point no longer be permitted. In the meantime, it has to be declared on the label. Beef 'previously frozen' and then minced should be labelled as such, but if it is mixed in with fresh beef it doesn't have to be.

Additives in beef products

A wide range of additives is common in cheaper beef products. These can include rusk (dried bread) to bind, water to bulk out, polyphosphates to retain added water, soya and milk proteins to bulk out and add texture, antioxidants to prevent rancidity and extend shelf life, colourings, flavour enhancers and seasonings, nitrates and nitrites (see page 137) and sugar.

As with all processed food, it pays to read the label very carefully. The fewer ingredients, the better. Acceptable additions include rusk and seasonings … it's downhill for quality and flavour thereafter.

AVOIDING FOOD POISONING FROM BEEF

A food poisoning bug, *E coli*, is responsible for large numbers of food poisoning cases each year. The risk is mostly associated with **beefburgers** that have been cooked from frozen but not cooked thoroughly enough right through to the centre of the burger to kill off the bugs. Of course, this bug should not be in the meat in the first place but as explained above, minced beef products are not exactly a high-quality food category! Another dubious item found both in local butcher's and in supermarkets, **flash-fry steak**, sounds more upmarket. Butchers now have the equipment to tenderise meat by passing it though a machine which inserts fine needles into it. However, this tenderising process may transfer any harmful bacteria that would normally be on the outside of the meat into the centre. This means that they are not killed off with quick grilling as they would be with normal steak. Ask your butcher or supermarket how their beef is tenderised. If this system is used, don't eat their flash-fry steak rare.

IS BEEF SAFE TO EAT?

Ever since the first cases of 'mad cow disease' or Bovine
Spongiform Encephalopathy (BSE) were noted in 1986,
there has been a question mark over the safety of beef.
Nothing has happened to give beef a clean bill of health
in the meantime and there are still grounds for keeping
it on your 'high-risk' list. Why?

Initially the government said that the source of the
disease was animal feed concentrates, contaminated with
the remains of sheep suffering from a disease called
scrapie. In 1988 the feeding of animal proteins to cattle,
sheep and deer (though not pigs and poultry) was
banned. Assuming that it had established the cause of the
problem and dealt with it, the government's Southwood
Committee predicted that cattle would be a 'dead-end
host' and that the disease would die out with all the cattle
that had eaten infected feed. It said that the risk to human
health was 'remote' and dismissed the possibility that the
disease could be passed on from cow to calf, or to other
species. It is now obvious that the government's experts
were wrong. Similar spongiform encephalopathies have
been found in other animal species, and there are claims
of human casualties from the human equivalent of BSE –
CJD (Creutzfeld Jakob disease). The disease has not died
out as it should have, boosting the theory that there is
transmission from cow to calf.

So where does that leave the consumer? We still do
not know the cause of the disease, the exact nature of
the 'infectious agent', and cannot predict how it will
evolve. Some independent experts say that it may be possible for humans to catch CJD from eating beef. They
point out that although obviously infected cattle are
put down, most beef cattle are slaughtered before the age

of two years and the signs of BSE appear only in much older animals. Also, beef from European surplus stocks, or 'intervention beef', which pre-dates the controls on feedstuffs and the sale of certain offals, is still being released on to the market. The worry is that beef from infected animals is passing into the human food chain undetected. If true, this means that a future epidemic of the equivalent of BSE in humans cannot be ruled out.

For the concerned consumer, there are some obvious precautions to be taken:

- The extreme reaction – stop eating beef.
- The compromise – eat only beef from beef-suckler herds (less than 15 per cent of beef-suckler herds have had BSE cases, while over 50 per cent of dairy herds have been affected).
- Only buy meat pies, sausages, burgers and so on from butchers or small suppliers who can guarantee that it comes from traditional beef herds.

Veal

Veal – the meat from milk-fed calves – can be marvellous, like eating sweet suckling pig or tender baby lamb. Most of the time, though, it is dry and flavourless. Why? Because it has been produced in a totally unnatural manner which is cruel to the calves. So if you eat veal, be quite clear about what you are getting.

THE BEST VEAL

This comes from calves that have been kept with their mothers and suckled by them, their diet supplemented by a little grass towards the end. Depending on the time of year, these calves will either be outdoors (in summer), or kept inside in family groups (in winter) in comfortable, spacious barns with generous beddings of straw.

This traditional way of rearing veal, most common in France where it is called '*veau sous la mère*', produces wonderful meat with a slightly pink hue. This is because the calf derives all the natural goodness it needs from its mother's milk and is kept in stress-free circumstances where it can exercise properly.

Very little veal is produced in this way, especially in the UK, where veal production is extremely limited anyway. When available, such meat sells for a premium price. Veal fed on mother's milk should come with a detailed guarantee, such as the French '*label rouge – veau sous la mère*', or from small-scale farmers who can tell you exactly how the calf was raised.

THE WORST VEAL

This is from calves that are taken away from their mothers, although separation is known to be stressful for both mother and calf, and then fed on a diet of milk powder made up with water, deficient in the nutrients found in natural mother's milk. This all-milk diet allows the farmer to produce meat that is white in colour but means that the calf is kept in a state of anaemia and the development of its stomach system is completely distorted.

Veal calves come from the dairy herd and are then sold via livestock markets. Many calves (including British ones) destined for veal production are exported by road for long distances, often arriving at their final destination dehydrated, starving, injured and, at the very least, stressed.

Thereafter, the calves are kept entirely indoors, never going outdoors to graze. In the cruellest system – now outlawed in Britain but common in Holland, France and Italy – the calves are kept in crates. These are small crates with slatted floors, no straw, where the calf does not have the space to turn around and cannot even stand up or lie down without difficulty.

This sort of veal production is extremely cruel. Besides the humanitarian arguments against it, the artificial feeding and indoor captivity of the calves makes for flavourless meat. Continental veal production of this kind has also been tainted by scandals, as evidence regularly comes to light showing that the use of illegal growth-promoting, beta-agonist drugs is surprisingly common.

Most imported veal is produced in this way. Unless the label explicitly states otherwise, you can assume that it is crated veal.

SLIGHTLY BETTER VEAL?

One slight improvement on the veal crate described above is the 'loose-house' system. Here, calves are still kept indoors but in barns or larger pens, where they can move around. Some loose-house systems have straw and bedding to give the calves more comfort and to satisfy their need to chew fibrous material. The ability to chew means that the calves do pick up more vitamins and trace elements from hay, which gives the meat a slightly pinker hue than crated veal. Some loose-house systems also permit animal-feed concentrates to be fed to the calves, which can produce even darker meat. Concentrates, however, are not necessarily an improvement on powdered milk because they can contain a number of undesirable additives (see page 114).

Not all the loose-house systems provide straw. Sometimes the calves are just left on concrete or slatted floors, even though the crate is not used, and there are no improvements in other ways. Nearly anything is better than the veal crate, but even in the best loose-house systems, the calves never go outdoors and are deprived of their mother's milk, making for unhappy animals and tasteless meat.

A little Dutch veal and most English veal is produced in this way. Labels promising more humane or welfare-conscious meat (in supermarkets and upmarket butchers) usually go on veal from this system, unless they specifically list other guarantees, such as that the calf was kept with its mother or allowed outdoors.

Lamb

If you want meat that is reasonably naturally produced and flavoursome, lamb is a good bet. Unlike pork and poultry, it does not lend itself to factory farming.

AN OUTDOOR LIFE

Sheep live outdoors, free to wander over large expanses, and are brought in to large, relatively open shelters for protection in extreme, harsh weather and at lambing time. Although it is possible to rear sheep indoors it is extremely uneconomic, so nearly all sheep are reared outdoors for most of their lives.

It is now possible to manipulate the sheep's reproductive cycle to make ewes breed out of season (see page 125). This goes hand in hand with indoor rearing but fortunately very few sheep are farmed in this way so far. On the whole, sheep remain stubbornly unproductive – giving birth just once a year – so they are of relatively low value to the farmer. As a result, it is actually cheaper to keep sheep in a very traditional way.

A WHOLESOME DIET

The natural lifestyle and diet of sheep show up in flavoursome meat. Upland sheep graze on heather, bracken and wild pasture, lowland sheep on sweet, lush grass and clover or salt marshes. The lamb takes on a particular flavour according to the type of feeding available. Most sheep come indoors for part of the winter, where they are fed on natural foods such as hay, silage (preserved grass) and crushed barley. It is not usual for this feed to be medicated, as is the case with other farm animals. Most sheep are routinely vaccinated against a number of different parasites, so you cannot assume that lamb is medicine or 'additive' free. However, all vaccinations should be carried out long before slaughter and traces should not be present in the meat.

One very controversial practice is dipping sheep in highly toxic organophosphorus chemicals to stop them getting infestations. This is a hazardous measure for the farmer, since exposure is linked to serious illness, and there is some concern over the impact these waste chemicals have when dumped. There is no evidence to suggest that the chemicals persist in the meat. Farmers have to observe strict withdrawal times between dipping and slaughter.

THE WELFARE OF SHEEP

When it comes to diet and exercise, sheep have a much better life than most farm animals. Any suffering tends to come in the form of neglect. Quite a high percentage (10–15 per cent) of lambs are thought to die out on the hills and in remote locations through cold and hunger.

Two mutilations are commonly carried out on sheep. The majority of male lambs are castrated by a variety of methods, and lambs of both sexes have part of their tail removed, or 'docked'. Most of these mutilations are carried out without anaesthetic and are known to cause pain and discomfort. Animal welfarists say that neither mutilation is routinely necessary and should only be carried out under anaesthetic by a vet. Many farmers insist that tail docking is necessary to protect the sheep from parasites which would cause them to suffer, and any pain caused is temporary.

Transport and slaughter of sheep has been another major cause for concern. A series of documented scandals, both in the UK and abroad, have highlighted the often disgracefully cruel handling of sheep and lambs, resulting in frequent deaths and casualties. Documented reports have witnessed rough handling and incorrect pre-stunning of sheep so that the animals may still be conscious when slaughtered. There is quite a lot of evidence to suggest that a proportion of sheep end their generally agreeable lives in great pain and suffering.

For the welfare-minded consumer, it is really very hard to discover the circumstances of slaughter. If you cannot buy lamb from the farmer direct, the best guarantee is to buy from independent butchers with a good reputation who can tell you exactly where their lamb comes from and where it has been slaughtered, or from large supermarket chains selling better-quality lamb. Neither of these has anything to gain from selling lamb that has been badly handled or slaughtered, since the stress suffered by the animal is likely to show up in tough, low-quality meat.

WHEN BRITISH LAMB IS IN SEASON

Spring lamb appears in shops anytime from March on. This is usually English lamb from milder, lowland pastures and is followed in the summer (June to September) by mainly Welsh and Scottish lamb, plus hill lamb from colder Northern English areas. A good butcher should be able to tell you which type of meat you are buying, and some new labels are appearing which stipulate the geographical origins, such as 'Scottish hill lamb'.

Unless it is imported (see page 126), **new-season lamb** available outside these periods is likely to come from the small number of indoor-kept sheep. The ewes will have been given hormones and kept inside under controlled lighting to make them breed out of season and produce more twins. By this means, farmers can sell them for a premium by offering new lamb when it would not otherwise be on the market. Encouragingly, relatively little lamb is produced in this way.

Spring or summer lamb should be small in size, with a pale, more tender flesh, a little less fat and a sweeter flavour, though this will vary according to the breed (see page 127).

As the autumn arrives, the sheep get bigger and the lamb will be stronger in flavour, slightly firmer and fattier in flesh. This **winter lamb** or just plain 'lamb', is known as **hogget** once it is more than a year old. Sheep that are over two years old can be sold as **mutton**, though very few are. A great pity, since slow-cooked mutton can be a very fine traditional delicacy.

JUDGING THE QUALITY OF LAMB

When you are buying spring lamb, look for deep-pink meat which is nicely marbled with pearly-white fat. More mature 'winter' lamb will be dark red with more marbling of fat, which will be creamier in colour. All the cuts should be neat and well butchered. That means nice even-sized chops and joints, with the 'fell' (the outer layer of skin) trimmed off and the bones free of excessive fat.

IMPORTED LAMB

Imported lamb from New Zealand has complementary seasons to our own. A certain amount of it is sold fresh and chilled, usually in the period between December and May when British spring lamb is scarce. Most New Zealand lamb, however, is sold frozen, and is spring lamb from sheep killed at six months. New Zealand lamb used to have a reputation for toughness, due to crude freezing. A more sophisticated technique has changed this so, despite being frozen, the lamb does taste rather good as well as being reliably tender. The cheaper price tag does not reflect inferior quality. Consumers prefer fresh chilled meat, and so there is a limit to what can be charged for frozen. Plus there are an awful lot of sheep in New Zealand!

In welfare terms, these sheep are kept even more extensively than most British sheep, and never indoors. In all other ways – vaccination, mutilations and so on – they are reared like British sheep.

ORGANIC LAMB

Organic sheep are reared in a similar way to conventional ones but will have grazed on pastures certified as organic – that is, they have not been treated with chemicals (see page 284). The organic guarantee is less important for upland and hill sheep, which tend to feed on untreated pastures anyway, but conventionally farmed lowland sheep may well graze on pasture that has been chemically treated. Organic sheep, on the other hand, are raised in naturally lush pastures and this should be reflected in the flavour of the lamb.

In some respects, animal welfare is superior for organic sheep. The amount of space allocated to sheep wintering indoors is more generous, permanent indoor rearing is not allowed and permitted journey time to slaughter is only eight hours. But they may still be tail docked (though not routinely) for animal welfare reasons. Organophosphorus sheep dips are banned.

THE BEST-TASTING BREEDS

Although lamb is generally a flavoursome meat, certain traditional breeds are thought to be specially good to eat. This reputation is partly to do with the breed but also due to the pasture with which these breeds are traditionally associated. Despite their geographical connections, such breeds can be produced in different types of environments the world over, with varying results.

Romney Marsh sheep used to be reared only in Kent but, now crossed with other breeds, it is the most common variety in New Zealand. Some Romney Marsh sheep are still produced in the eponymous marshland. It is a favourite breed for salty, coastal pastures which are thought to give the meat a special character. **Soay, Scottish Blackface, Shetland** and **Welsh Mountain** sheep are all very old breeds, developed for their hardiness, which are thought to have a particularly good flavour, being slightly gamier and darker fleshed.

Some butchers will be able to tell you the breed of their lamb but not many can because they buy through intermediaries. Most butchers should nevertheless be able to tell you the geographical area from which the lamb came, which is a rough guide to the type of breed. Hill lamb, for example, is more likely to be a hardy, traditional breed. Some useful supermarket labels are appearing, such as 'Scottish or Welsh hill lamb'.

Pork – including sausages, ham, bacon, salami and pâté

Pork is a perfect symbol of both the excesses of modern intensive-production methods and the farming industry's ability to change when under consumer pressure. Amongst all our farm animals, the intelligent and sociable pig has suffered some of the worst indignities and deprivations. In the natural order of things, a pig would spend most of its time outside foraging in woodland or rooting around a field. With the arrival of modern animal-production systems, it was brought into densely packed sheds, separated from its family group and fed high-protein food of dubious origins to obtain ever-more ambitious production rates. Ten years ago, it would have been extremely difficult to find pork that had not been raised in this sort of system.

Encouragingly, there has been something of a consumer-led revolution in pork production over the last few years. This is because the eating quality had become so bad – tough, watery, tasteless – and the conditions of the animals so notorious, that an industry rethink became necessary. Outdoor pork, which had previously been written off by agricultural advisors as 'uneconomic', was pioneered on a large commercial scale by Marks and Spencer in the late 1980s and now 20 per cent of British pork production comes from outdoor systems. Vigorous campaigning by animal welfare groups has resulted in legislation to phase out the infamous 'sow stall' – where sows spent all their time unable to turn around and often tethered – by 1999. An estimated 300,000 to 350,000 British pigs are still kept in these at present.

More than half the bacon consumed on mainland Britain comes from Ireland, Holland and Denmark, where sow stalls are still the dominant system. If you care about animal welfare, boycott Danish, Dutch and Irish pork. Don't have any illusions that British ham and bacon production is perfect either; it is just better in this minimum respect.

Recent improvements mean that there is absolutely no need to settle for old-style indoor pork, ham or bacon. Any supermarket or independent butcher worth its salt should be able to offer you pork that comes from an outdoor system. This sort of pork is the most humane, and much more likely to taste good.

JUDGING THE QUALITY OF PORK

Nice fresh pork should be pale pink and have a slight sheen to it. Thereafter, there are certain visual signs indicating poor meat that will not eat well. Some pork is known as having PSE – short for pale, soft, exudative flesh. As the title suggests, this is meat that looks paler than usual, is floppy and does not seem to hold its shape. It will look wet and produce quite a lot of fluid in the pack or wrapper. Another set of faults is DFD – short for dark, firm, and dry. Though pork should not drip too much, a little moisture is quite normal. It shouldn't, however, be too dry either.

THE BEST-TASTING BREEDS

The most common British pig is the **Large White** crossed with the **Duroc**. It has been bred for its leanness and its ability to grow quickly – the key industry objectives. Many consumers and butchers now believe that, for flavour and texture, these modern pigs cannot compare with our more traditional breeds, such as the

Berkshire, the Tamworth, the Gloucestershire Old Spot and the British Saddleback. Unlike their more commercial counterparts, these breeds are fattier, take longer to mature and are better adapted to outdoor production. Whether it is because of the breed or the way they are produced is debatable, but farmers rearing these breeds are likely to be offering the best pork available.

THE WORST PORK

The majority of British pigs still live their lives indoors, in miserable circumstances. They are kept in a series of small pens on hard concrete or slatted floors. The pregnant sows are separated from the rest of their family group a day or two before labour and kept in what are known as farrowing crates, very similar to sow stalls. The sow spends around four weeks in these just before and after birth, and is unable to turn around. The reason given for this is that the sow would otherwise crush her piglets, an argument which many animal welfarists and vets hotly dispute. They believe it just makes management easier for the farmer. In natural circumstances, the sow would make a comfortable bed out of straw and select a spot for giving birth.

In order to get the maximum productivity out of each sow, the piglets are separated from their mother – early weaning – at about four weeks, which is much earlier than they would if left to themselves. This means that the sow can be re-mated earlier and produce yet another litter. The modern pig has been bred to produce larger and larger litters and the standard litter now consists of 10 to 12 piglets, where it used to be four to five. New breeds of 'super sow' have even been bred to have 18 teats, instead of the usual 12, so they can feed even more piglets. The standard British sow produces on average five litters of about 11 piglets in two years, while normally she would produce only two or three. After two years, most sows are so worn out with the strain of constant pregnancies that they are slaughtered, their meat destined for low-grade sausages.

The piglets have their teeth clipped to prevent them damaging their littermates as they compete for teats.

These piglets, which are taken away from their mothers prematurely for separate fattening, often behave in an abnormal way, still trying to suck and nose. One substitute for their mother would be some straw or bedding. Pigs love straw, not just for the comfort but for its playing potential. They also like playing around with old rubber tyres and so on. But in most intensive systems, bedding and other diversions are not provided and so the piglets become heartily bored with being kept in a barren environment. This is when they start fighting with each other and nibbling at each others' tails. The standard response to this is to 'dock' or cut off their tails, an unnecessary mutilation which is a direct consequence of the conditions in which they are kept.

The diet of the indoor pig is radically different from the fresh green food and forage roots it would eat in natural circumstances. Most factory-farm pigs are fed on pelleted rations bought in from feed-compounder companies. The bulk of it is cereal and/or another carbohydrate such as whey but it usually also contains a higher protein element. This can be something acceptable such as soya, but it can legally also be fish meal, animal by-products (meat, feather meals), and dry poultry manure (recycled carcasses and feathers).

Antibiotics and probiotics are routinely given in feed to keep the diseases endemic to intensive farming at bay. There is evidence to suggest that withdrawal periods from antibiotics are not always observed, since residues in pork for human consumption turn up from time to time in spot checks. This could have serious consequences for human health as strains of antibiotics may become so common in animals, and thus the human gut, that they become medically useless. Copper supplements are also included to speed up growth.

Unless the label explicitly states otherwise, you can assume that pork, ham and bacon come from this system.

BETTER PORK

This comes from outdoor, or free-range, pigs who at least have experienced a period of outdoor life at some point in their existence. Normally the breeding sow and boar live outdoors in fields where they can forage, returning to movable arcs, bedded with straw, for warmth and comfort. The sows will not give birth in a farrowing crate. So far so good.

Thereafter systems differ. In the best systems the piglets will also remain outdoors, but often they will be weaned early from their mothers and put inside to fatten in barns. The circumstances of these vary according to the farmer. Some barns are light, warm and airy, and generously bedded with straw – creature comforts the pigs appreciate. Because they have more to do and play with, the piglets do not need to be routinely tail docked or tooth clipped. Routine medication of feed is usually, but not necessarily, prohibited in favour of selective treatment of ailing animals.

However, there is no legal definition of outdoor pork, so the piglets for fattening may equally be transferred into gloomy, factory-farm sheds, like their intensive counterparts, and suffer the same deprivations. Most outdoor pork is nevertheless a vast improvement on indoor intensive pork, in terms of both animal welfare and eating quality. A commitment to some form of outdoor production shows that the farmer is at least interested in doing better.

Outdoor pork of some description is now available in most supermarket chains, from the best independent butchers and direct or by mail order from producers. Such pork is always labelled 'outdoor-bred' to distinguish it from run-of-the-mill pork, and often accompanied by an explanatory leaflet.

ORGANIC PORK

The production of organic pigs is everything that intensive indoor pork is not. Outdoor production is the norm but under certain limited circumstances indoors is permitted – at least for part of the pig's life. When indoors, the pigs must be kept in warm, ventilated sheds, well bedded with straw and provided with 'toys' so that they can play and amuse themselves without becoming aggressive. Farrowing crates for sows are not permitted and neither is early weaning – piglets must not be taken away from their mother before six weeks and usually at eight weeks. The pigs are kept in small, stable groups and tail docking, routine tooth cutting and castration are all banned. Antibiotics, probiotics and copper for growth promotion are not permitted, and commercial compound feeds are banned. Feed and swill must come from a restricted list of acceptable natural foodstuffs, excluding all dubious animal sources, monitored by the Soil Association. At least 70 per cent of the diet must come from organic sources and 60 per cent must be made from fresh green food or unmilled forage. When outdoors, the pigs root around on organic land that has not been treated with chemicals.

Organic pork is becoming more widely available and is best bought direct from the producer. A list of producers is available from the Soil Association (see page 292).

'FREEDOM FOOD' PORK

This RSPCA-approved label promises much in welfare terms but is curiously disappointing. Outdoor production is not required or even emphasised, while farrowing crates, tail docking and tooth clipping are all allowed. Freedom Food pigs can eat the same diet as intensive, indoor pigs including food from animal sources, antibiotics and other additives previously described.

Improvements guaranteed by this label include straw for bedding and a journey limit time for transport of live pigs. All in all, this label is not even as good as the most basic forms of free-range, outdoor pork, and only a marginal improvement on indoor intensive pork.

PORK SAUSAGES

If you want good-quality pork, sausages are least likely to offer it. Obviously there are exceptions, and there has been a recent surge of interest in the banger which is very positive. Specialist shops are opening up and many of these produce quite good sausages from good-quality meat, which are happily free from the additives listed below. However, sausage labelling, both in supermarkets and small shops, is full of descriptions such as 'traditional', 'old-style', 'original' and so on which are totally unregulated. Don't take them as a guarantee of quality. When buying sausages you need to know the quality of the basic meat (whether it is standard indoor pig, free-range or organic), and then have a good look at the label.

The quality of the basic meat

Meat products are covered by a legal 'minimum meat declaration'. To call itself a pork sausage, a product must contain only 65 per cent pork. But don't make the mistake of presuming that this is from prime cuts. Meat in these products can come from several sources, including meat scraps from trimmed carcasses, parts of the animal most consumers don't want (tail meat, head meat, cheek, neck, shin, tongue, kidney, gristle, sinew), fat (up to 50 per cent), fatty cuts (belly, flank), pork from tired-out old sows, frozen imported pork, and mechanically recovered, or mechanically separated meat (MRM).

MRM is under review by the European Commission and may at some point no longer be permitted. In the meantime, it has to be declared on the label. Otherwise, the exact make-up of the pork used does not need to be declared. Some mass-manufactured 'value' and 'economy' lines contain as little as 50 per cent meat, which is usually an unsavoury blend of low-grade poultry meat, pork and beef. Don't touch them with a bargepole.

Additives in pork sausages

Like beef, cheaper pork products contain a wide range of additives. These can include: rusk – dried wheat bread (to bind), water (to bulk out), polyphosphates (to retain added water), soya and milk proteins (to bulk out and add texture), antioxidants (to prevent rancidity and extend shelf life), colourings, flavour enhancers and seasonings both natural and synthetic, nitrates and nitrites (see page 137) to give a pink colour and to preserve, and sugar.

When you buy processed pork products, read the ingredients list very carefully and choose ones that contain as few ingredients as possible. If you buy sausages from your local butcher, ingredients are even less prominently on display. Quiz your butcher about what goes into them.

FINDING DECENT HAM AND BACON

Ham and bacon is cured (salt-preserved) pork. Ham should be the hind leg of the pig, while bacon can come from other parts – back, belly, neck and so on.

A good ham should be moist and meltingly soft to the bite. Bacon should sizzle away in the pan and produce no water or white liquid. Eventually the fat should brown and crisp up beautifully.

The telltale signs that all is not well are only too familiar. In bacon, a horrible white liquid oozes out of the rashers and the fat refuses to crisp up. In ham, you can see a sheen to the meat, and in the mouth it often has a slippery, unyielding texture reminiscent of Spam.

The succulence of decent cooked ham and the crispness of a good bacon rasher are both a direct result of how it has been cured. Traditionally there are two different methods: **dry salting**, where the pork is coated with salt and seasonings, then left to sit until it is cured; and **brine**, where the pork is left in a salty soaking liquid until it is cured.

Some specialist bacon curers, organic and small-scale pork farmers still produce their hams and bacons by these methods. However, most modern ham and bacon is cured in a highly industrial process which is a development of the brining method. Machines with a series of very fine needles inject the meat with the brine solution, which is made up of water mixed with salt and various preservatives – nitrites and nitrates (see page 137). Polyphosphates, an additive that helps the meat retain water (and thus weigh more heavily), are routinely incorporated into the brine solution. This means that the pork can be cured much more quickly and profitably for the manufacturer.

Modern ham, unlike traditional ham which was always made from the hind leg of the pig, is often re-formed by taking bits of meat from other parts of the pig, massaging, tumbling and then pressing them together into easy-to-slice blocks or rounds. In the process, water is added, as well as other additives such as sugar, gelatine, yeast extract and hydrolised vegetable protein. These either help to hold it together or give it some flavour.

Some smoked bacon is not smoked over wood at all but sprayed with a synthetic flavouring product known in the trade as liquid smoke, on the same principle as 'bacon-flavour crisps'. Liquid smoke is widely used throughout the industry, although many bacon curers do have their own smokehouses. There is no legal requirement to define by what method bacon is smoked and therefore there is no obligation to state on the label that liquid smoke has been used. One way to avoid liquid smoke is to buy ham and bacon that says 'smoked over oak chips', 'traditionally smoked' or something to that effect.

UK regulations allow up to 10 per cent of the weight of ham and bacon to be made up of water without it being declared on the label. If it contains more water than this, it has to be declared. Don't be taken in by labels that say 'not more than 15 per cent added water'. This means that they could contain up to 25 per cent added water! Usually, the more water in a 'ham', the more additives too. Needless to say, this hi-tech approach is no improvement on traditional methods and produces water-logged, poor-value meat.

- Brine-cured bacon and ham are best avoided in favour of dry-cured. All supermarkets stock a dry-cured line (often sold as 'traditionally cured'), as do good independent butchers. Small specialist suppliers nearly all prefer to dry-cure their hams and bacon.

- If you cannot find dry-cured, buy meat that says 'no added water' – even then it may include 10 per cent.

- When given the choice with cooked hams, opt for one that has been carved from the bone on the spot, since it is more likely to have been cured in a more natural way. Avoid tinned ham – it's the worst quality around.

- Look carefully at the ham and avoid any that are obviously made up from re-formed bits. If you have to buy de-boned, de-fatted and de-rinded ham, buy slices from one joint, such as loin.

- Be suspicious of shiny hams which glisten in the way that petrol does when mixed with water. These are highly adulterated. Good natural ham should look pale pink and have a slightly matt surface.

- Be suspicious of 'economy' bacon lines. These are most likely to use liquid smoke (see above).

PRESERVATIVES IN CURED MEATS

Nitrites and nitrates are routinely used in modern curing. They have the effect of dehydrating the pork and inhibiting the growth of bacteria, thus preserving the meat. They also give the ham or bacon its stable pink colour. There is a long-running debate as to the safety of these preservatives, which are known carcinogens in animals.

It is probably the case that they have been overused in the past, and recently the permitted amounts have been reduced. They are already banned in baby food.

Some people think they are unnecessary, dangerous, and used only for the food manufacturer's advantage, while others argue that preservatives are an important safeguard against food poisoning such as botulism. It is probably not a good idea to eat excessive quantities of cured meats. Favour products containing no more than two, and preferably just one, of the preservatives listed below. Some bacon, for example, contains salt and two or three different preservatives when only one would do.

Suspect nitrites and nitrates:

- Potassium nitrite E249
- Sodium nitrite E250
- Sodium nitrate E251
- Potassium nitrate E252

'PRODUCT OF THE UK' – A MEANINGLESS TITLE

Anything can be described as 'Product of the UK' providing it has been 'substantially changed' there. Thus it is legal to sell bacon or ham as 'product of the UK' if that is where it was cured. It does not mean that the pigs themselves have been raised in the UK. Sometimes Danish, Dutch or even Irish pigs are exported to the UK where they are turned into 'British' bacon. This allows curers and supermarket chains to take advantage of price fluctuations but still cash in on 'Buy British' loyalties. The **'Charter-Quality British Bacon' logo** – a small British Isles symbol – can only appear on bacon from pigs reared and cured in Britain, and the blue **'Quality-Assured Scottish Pork' logo** can only be used for home-produced pigs. A British bacon label in itself is no guarantee of British pork.

BACON AND HAM TALK TRANSLATED

Bacon usually comes from parts of the pig other than the hind legs. **Back, oyster, collar** and **streaky** all refer to cuts of bacon. Unsmoked bacon can be called **green** or **pale**. **Pancetta** is the Italian equivalent of bacon. **Gammon** is the name for the hind leg of a bacon pig after curing. When cooked, it is usually called **ham**. **Gammon rashers** or **steaks** are cut from the hind leg.

York ham is the traditional mild English ham, taken from the hind leg of the pig which is unsmoked. **Bradenham ham** is a variation which, after sweet-curing, is pickled in molasses and juniper to give it a black skin. **Alderton ham** is lightly smoked and roasted in a marmalade glaze.

Wiltshire is just the name for the most common type of British cure, where whole sides are cured, skin on. **Ayrshire** cure is similar, but the meat is skinned and boned first. **Suffolk** is a traditional British sweet cure. Bacon sold as **sweet, mild** or **tender** cure has had some sweetener added to the brine.

Sliced cooked ham and pork liver pâté – be very choosy

If you fancy courting food poisoning, then look no further than the deli. Ready-sliced ham, sold loose, is one of the most common vehicles for food-poisoning bacteria such as salmonella, listeria and staphylococcus aureus. Spot checks carried out in the UK by the Consumers' Association have shown that around 80 per cent of samples of sliced ham bought from delicatessens were contaminated. Small butchers, and supermarket deli counters were a little better, with 'only' around 40 per cent contaminated.

When you cannot buy ham sliced from the bone on the spot, ham sliced and sold in pre-packs is probably safer than loose.

Pork pâtés are highly suspect, too. Apart form the usual strains of bacteria, mentioned above, which colonise them on the typical poorly maintained deli counter, residues of animal medicines – both legal and illegal – turn up in 'Brussels'-type pâtés with some regularity. Such pâtés are often sold with attractive titles – pork with pheasant, wild mushroom, country, and so on – and come in rustic-looking bowls. But they tend to contain a very high proportion of pork livers, which have concentrated residues of a wide gamut of undesirable drugs fed to pigs. Unless you like to live dangerously, pork liver of unknown pedigree should be off your shopping list – in all forms!

Hams eaten raw

Although Britain does not have a strong tradition of eating finely sliced raw cured ham, many countries in Europe do. The quality of the ham depends on a number of factors. First, there's the provenance of the pig, the way it has been raised and the quality of its feed. The pigs used for Parma ham, for example, are fed on the whey left over from the manufacture of parmigiano reggiano cheese, which is thought to lend them a distinctive flavour. Many Spanish and Portuguese pigs come from special breeds which root up acorns and beech mast in the forest, giving the meat a particular character. Second, there is the type of cure. Some are drycured with spices and salt, others in an aromatic salt brine to which elements such as wine are added. Then there is the patience with which the ham is dried, which can vary from artisanal to totally hi-tech methods. Finally, if the ham is smoked, the method of smoking (traditional smokehouse or modern kiln) and the smoking medium (various types of wood, such as hickory, oak or spruce, or even peat) make a difference.

These days there are many different types of ham on the market and price is generally the best guide to quality. The finest raw hams all have their cheaper copies, and confusion in translation – genuine or deliberate – leaves room for consumer deception.

Unlike sliced cooked ham, raw hams are cured and matured

in such a way that they last for months and even years without refrigeration. This means that, as a general rule, they do not present the same food-safety problems.

The Italians favour an unsmoked melt-in-the-mouth style of ham, with a delicate balance of flavour between salt and meat. When buying **Italian** hams, look out for **Parma** ham bearing a crown logo with the words 'Genuine Parma ham'. **San Danielle** and **Culatello** are arguably even finer but they cost more and are not widely available. **Prosciutto** is just a word for cured ham (or even just plain pork in Italy) and cheaper copies of Parma ham are often sold with this name. They can taste fine, if not distinguished, but make sure you are not paying a Parma ham price for them! **Coppa** is not strictly a ham but cured pork neck, moulded into salami shape.

French hams, such as **Bayonne** and **Ardennes**, rarely match the finesse of the Italian ones. They are made in a chewier, leaner style, and usually served more thickly sliced. Buy ones bearing the French 'Label Rouge' quality mark. **German Black Forest** and **Westphalian** hams are firmer in the mouth and especially appreciated for their assertive smoky character. **Spanish Serrano** ham generally has a stronger, meatier flavour than Italian ham and more texture. Look out for Serrano ham with a *conzorzio* stamp (a teardrop shape with an 'S' in it) as a guarantee of quality. Some Serrano hams can look scrappier than Italian ones but this is just because they have not been moulded. Serranio **Iberico** is the name given to the finest hams, which come from traditional breeds of black pig fed on a very high-quality natural diet, usually acorns. **Portuguese Presunto** resembles the Serrano style, since the black pig, or *pata negra* breed, has its origins in Portugal. **British air-dried** hams are a bit of a novelty, and tend to be quite chewy.

Imported 'salamis' – a shopper's challenge

The French have their *charcuterie*, the Italians their *salami*. The UK, however, has no such tradition of cured, chopped meat, usually pork, stuffed into intestines and eaten raw. This makes us a captive audience for junk. The vast majority of imported cured 'salamis' we are asked to buy are of really poor quality. Unfamiliar as we are with this type of meat, we often do not know any better.

At its best, the process of making fine saucissons, salamis, and so on demands a lot of patience and is nothing short of an art. Salamis are just cured meat – a mixture of lean and fat – which is pre-salted, rested, chopped to various degrees of coarseness or fineness depending on the recipe, cured, rested again, then stuffed into natural animal intestines and matured until quite dry.

The provenance of the base meat, the curing technique, and the manner in which it is matured all play a part. Unfortunately, most modern salamis are industrial copies of the real thing, and the worst examples are just bargain-basement Danish or German copies of the industrial copies. Even illustrious names – such as Jésus de Lyon, saucisson d'Arles, Felino and Milano – once guarantees of quality, are no longer dependable. There are very few really high-quality versions about and only a tiny number of them are imported to the UK. The majority of salamis we see on our shelves have been made by fast-track methods. Pork, but sometimes beef, is bought by large curers. This should be the traditional hind leg of pork but often cheaper bits such as head and shin are included. Both lean and fat are bought in frozen. The meat is cut up quickly by machine, instead of by hand, which means that tougher bits that were previously unusable, such as tendon and nerve, can be incorporated without seeming too tough.

The traditional cures of salt, pepper, some aromatics and perhaps alcohol are replaced by modern brines, which include sugar, polyphosphates, acids, colourings and flavour enhancers all designed to make the meat look good and have a long sell-by date. They also help stabilise the excess water from the frozen meat. Natural casings or intestines have been supplanted by ones made from 'animal collagen', which is glued-together guts, tendon and soluble skin. A flour is used so they appear to have the natural 'bloom' that occurs on well-matured salamis. A rapid drying follows, allowing the finished salami to be on the shelf in weeks, not the months of its traditional equivalent.

Most salamis produced in this way are very unsavoury concoctions which are sold cheaply and anonymously. If your head throbs and you feel dehydrated after a salami-type lunch, your body is reacting to the onslaught of chemical additives.

Amongst the least savoury are the salamis that producers have the nerve to call low fat. These claims are not regulated. Many 'low-fat' salamis contain more fat than the authentic original version would, but the impression of leanness is given by mincing the fat more finely through the lean, so consumers do not see cubes of fat. The truth is that all salamis are relatively high-fat food, although there is no obligation for curers to list the fat content on the label.

Labels on salamis tend to be coy in the extreme, devoid of any useful information. In the face of any hard information to the contrary, it pays to think the worst! So:

- Choose Italian, Spanish or French salamis and buy the most expensive you can find in each category (Napoli, Chorizo, Rosette and so on). Favour those few that come with some pedigree (breed, feed, maturation process, brief, clear additives listing).
- Favour salamis in natural casings that are not of uniform diameter (irregular shape, thinner at the ends, with string well stuck on to the casing). These are likely to be less industrial.
- Buy salamis that are salami-shaped (described above), not square, trapezoid or with funny faces in the middle. These are all marketing gimmicks and do not bode well for the basic quality.
- Avoid Danish and German salamis. These are usually entirely industrial, surprisingly fatty, additive-laden and excessively salty.
- Be wary of 'Hungarian' salami. This term is now used as a style, rather than a country of origin. Most salami sold under this title is of the Danish and German type.
- Boycott low-fat salamis – they tend to be additive-laden as well as dishonest.

- Give a wide berth to anything that looks like Spam. This type of sausage is made from a low-grade frankfurter-type mix of pork slurry and chemical additives.
- Avoid lurid colours. Darker terracotta chorizos, for example, are more authentic than bright pinky-orange ones. These contain inferior paprika and artificial colours. Bad Danish salamis give themselves away with a colour more appropriate to raspberries than cured meat.

Game

In theory, game is the ultimate in natural meat, coming from animals that have lived in the wild, eating self-selected food appropriate to their species and exercising freely.

Would that it were that simple! Within the catch-all category of game, you'll find meat that lives up to your most romantic notion of wild food, meat that is half farmed, half wild, meat that is farmed in free-ranging circumstances, and meat that is as intensively produced as the average broiler chicken.

Wild game

You can safely put **hare, mallard duck, widgeon and teal, woodcock, snipe, plover and wood pigeon, partridge** and **grouse** in the category of truly wild game. These are not farmed. **Rabbit** and **deer** may be wild or farmed – you will need to ask. **Pheasant** is presumed wild but most of them start off life in commercial hatcheries (see below).

The pedigree of truly wild game is a bit of a mystery, and the quality of the meat itself can be very hit and miss. Game is only as wholesome as the countryside that supports it. Though certain areas, such as the north of Scotland, are still relatively rich in game and the habitat to sustain it, other areas are so transformed by the impact of intensive agriculture and industrial pollution that the environment of any remaining game is dramatically different. A wild deer, for example, may have been feeding on the traditional heather and roots or it may have strayed on to a field or forestry plantation recently sprayed with pesticides. There is no way of telling.

In animal welfare terms, although wild animals do not suffer any of the cruelty or deprivation associated with factory farming, you cannot assume automatically that they are healthy and thriving. Life can be tough out in the wild, with many animals struggling against the elements, unable to find adequate feeding, or affected by injury or disease.

Game can be one of the biggest treats you will ever eat, but the difficulty selecting it is that it is highly variable. Several factors affect the eating quality:

- the species of the animal (see page 147)
- its breeding status (lactating female deer, for example, are likely to be in poor condition; rutting stags or bucks have meat which is pale and smelly)
- the age of the animal (generally the older, the tougher and the more sinewy)
- its state of health (diseased, sickly, injured or malnourished animals should be avoided)
- the way it was shot (the best have been cleanly shot without making a mess of the carcass, because damage can travel quite a long way through the meat and produce an over-strong taste)
- how it has been bled (venison that has not been bled adequately, for example, will taste black and unpleasantly livery)
- how it has been handled (bruising adversely affects flavour)
- the way it has been matured (game which hasn't been hung may be tough and have little flavour; overhung game may taste too pungent).

THE TRICKY BUSINESS OF ASSESSING THE QUALITY OF WILD GAME

The eating quality of wild game rests on the factors above, and it takes an experienced eye to assess them. Even if you buy wild game from a butcher who specialises in it, it is not always easy to find out exactly what you are buying – where it came from, age, species, anticipated tenderness, and so on. Most butchers buy their game ready-prepared from a dealer. Game birds are usually plucked, without their beaks, feet and feathers, so it is not possible to age them. Larger game, such as deer, can only be aged by their teeth, but they come in minus their heads. These days, a lot of game supplied to butchers comes ready boned and diced.

If you buy supermarket wild game, the pedigree is no more obvious and you will just have to trust that the meat has been graded sensibly, which on the whole it is. Most supermarkets divide their wild game into categories such as roasting, stewing and grilling, which are fairly self-explanatory. The main problem is that it has rarely been hung and matured in the way a traditional game dealer might do, since most supermarkets have a horror of anything with a strong smell. Depending on your preference, some people find supermarket game underhung and lacking in flavour. But those who find some game a bit over the top often prefer it that way.

WILD GAME – THE BEST SPECIES

When it comes to wild venison, **roe deer** is often rated over **fallow, sika** or the more common **red deer** because it is a smaller animal and therefore has finer-grained flesh. Also, since roe deer do not live as long as other deer, the chances of getting a tender young roe are higher. **Grey-legged partridge** are leaner and taste better than **red-legged**. The **red** or **Scottish grouse** is said to taste better than (and substantially different from) black members of the grouse family such as **ptarmigan** and **capercaillie** but this is hard to prove, since such birds are relatively rare.

Extensively farmed and parkland game

Venison and wild boar come under this category.

Most farmed **deer** spend a large part of their lives grazing outdoors, except in winter when they are brought into large airy, straw-bedded barns and fed on a diet of root vegetables, hay and silage (preserved grass). One variation on deer farming is the parkland system. This is like farming but the deer have more space to roam over appropriate land, which has been fenced-in, and they are not usually brought in over winter or checked for disease.

Farmed venison has been developed in recent times as a highly welfare-conscious, free-range meat. The deer (mainly red deer) do not get pelleted rations or the routine medication of many farm animals.

Unlike wild deer, which are shot at a distance, farmed deer are shot at point-blank range in the field. This means that farmed venison is not affected by bullet damage, while wild venison nearly always is, and will not have that black livery flavour which comes from bruising and damage. Compared to other farm animals, deer do not experience any of the stress associated with transport to market or slaughterhouse. Guaranteed feeding, veterinary care when needed, and winter shelter all conspire to produce meat that is reliably tender, consistent and more likely to please than wild. One quality mark worth looking for when you are buying farmed venison is BPV – British Prime Venison – which guarantees that the deer is from accredited British farms. A lot of imported venison comes from New Zealand where welfare standards are lower (they remove the antlers to sell for oriental medicine and use routine medication).

Most supermarkets prefer their own guarantee, simply displaying the meat as 'Scottish' or 'English'.

There are two different sorts of **'wild boar'**: the real thing (pure-bred), which has usually been bred from imported wild boars, and cross-bred, from traditional breeds of pig such as the Tamworth which have been bred with imported wild boars. The first is leaner, darker and pleasantly chewy with a strong gamy flavour. The second is just like really good pork.

Wild boar meat is not very widely available but usually comes from free-range farmed, or parkland systems, on land that offers the pigs appropriate feeding – grass, scrub, bracken and so on – supplemented by root crops and potatoes. This makes for slow-growing animals and excellent meat. Like venison, wild boar has been developed by forward-thinking farmers as a wholesome and natural meat. Welfare standards are usually high: the pigs are kept in family groups, routine preventative medicine is out, and slaughter is carefully managed to minimise stress.

Half-farmed half-wild game: pheasant

Although pheasant is naturally a wild bird, most modern pheasants start their lives in similar circumstances to free-range chickens (see Chicken, Turkey and Other Farmed Poultry). The chicks are reared in hatcheries indoors and then gradually moved outdoors into yards with wire coops. During this time, because they are being kept in unnaturally densely packed circumstances, they are likely to have their beaks clipped to prevent aggression. They are fed on pelleted rations and given preventative medicines against parasites. Sometime before the season opens on 1 October, they are released so that they can fly off for shooting. Those that are promptly shot will taste little better than the most basic standard free-range chicken. The others that get away may enjoy a period of natural feeding and exercise, which means that they offer the eating qualities associated with pheasant in the wild. It's anyone's guess which you are getting when you buy one.

Farmed rabbit, quail and guinea fowl

Farmed **rabbit** are radically different from wild. They are usually reared entirely indoors, in small wire cages similar to battery cages for laying hens (see Chicken, Turkey and Other Farmed Poultry). The sheds are brightly lit to encourage regular breeding and high intake of food. The food in question is pelleted rations, which consist primarily of fish meal. More natural green foods and grains can be fed as a supplement, but whole diets like this are considered uneconomic because the rabbits do not grow quickly enough to make it 'commercial'. Deprived of any exercise and natural feeding, the rabbit is a miserable factory-farmed animal, with none of the notional virtues of game. Unless there is some indication on the label that farmed rabbit comes from a more humane system, assume the worst.

These days, **quail** and **guinea fowl** are always farmed (see pages 82 and 86).

Milk, Dairy Products and Cheese

The milk of dairy cows, together with all its derivative products, such as cream, cheese and butter, is a phenomenally important source of food. Milk has always had a generally good image in Britain as healthy and natural. However, it is increasingly the case that most of our milk is produced at great cost to the welfare of the dairy cow and to the environment. As a food, it is much altered from its 'natural' form by the time we consume it.

The welfare of dairy cows

The image of Daisy the contented cow is not quite as appropriate as it once was. The modern dairy cow has been selectively bred (see page 159) to be a prodigious milk machine, churning out greater volumes of milk than ever before. The metabolic pressure this puts on the cow is enormous. In the natural order of things, a cow would live until she was about 20. Nowadays, the average dairy cow is run like a machine on the edge of physiological breakdown – nine months in calf, nine months in milk, and six months both pregnant and lactating. As a result, most dairy cows have to be slaughtered before they are five years old – culled when their milk yield drops below 'economic' levels.

The size of the welfare problem is mirrored in the size of the modern cow. The drive for higher milk yields has encouraged the breeding of larger animals than ever before, with huge, bulging udders. The rest of the cow's anatomy has not kept pace with the 'improved' milking capacity. It is common for cows to suffer from such distended and heavy udders that they cannot walk properly and so often suffer from lameness. Mastitis – a painful infection of the udder – is quite common, exacerbated by over-production and frequent milking. Other common ailments include metabolic disorders such as milk fever, ketosis and staggers. All of these are strongly associated with the tremendous pressure placed on high-yielding cows.

Predictably, medication is often necessary in dairy herds. Mastitis, for example, is often treated automatically with anti-biotics, which will come out in the milk for a few days after treatment. Such milk should never be passed on for sale, and strict withdrawal periods should be observed. Antibiotic residues picked up in milk from time to time show that this is not always the case. Routine anthelmintics (anti-parasite drugs) are often standard procedure in large, intensive dairy herds, though in good farming practice treatment should be given only when there is a definite infestation, not on a preventative basis.

Diet has changed, too. The grass, roots and leafy forage that should form the bulk of the cow's diet have to be supplemented with high-protein foods in pelleted concentrates. These include various grains, soya beans, fish meal and animal waste, none of which is part of the cow's natural diet. Animal waste is highly suspect. Mad cow disease (BSE) is thought to have entered the dairy herd in this type of feed (see page 119).

This unnatural diet often causes gut upset and, in turn diarrhoea and leakage, which means that cows are often standing in dirt and wet. In addition, the increased feeding of silage (see below), means that the animals produce more liquid slurry. Since many cubicles constructed for cows only in the last few decades are already too small for the modern cow's back end and udders, they have to stand with their back legs in the pathways designed to collect slurry. Though most British cows spend their summers outdoors, in winter many pass most of the day tied up in cow-houses with slatted or solid concrete floors, with only a short exercise period. This puts even more pressure on their legs. In more humane systems, the cows are 'loose-housed' in groups inside more spacious yards, where they are also given straw for bedding.

Last but not least, after 40 weeks of pregnancy, at yearly intervals, the cow is separated from her calf on day one – a practice that is demonstrably upsetting for both cow and calf. Female calves provide the next generation of milkers. Male calves suited to beef production are sold for that purpose (see page 114), while others are sold for veal – usually in highly intensive circumstances (see page 121). As for the cow, it's off to the milking parlour two or three times a day.

Despite the fact that a European system of milk quotas (restrictions in production to control surplus) is still in operation, scientists are always looking for new ways to improve milk yield. The driving force is to get maximum yield out of a few very productive cows in intensive dairy herds. Animal welfarists and many consumers would be happier with more cows, lower yields and more humane milk production. A genetically engineered hormone called bovine somatotropin (BST) has been accepted for use on cows in the USA. This encourages better milk yields but puts the already stressed dairy cow under even more pressure.

Opposition from consumers, farmers and food retailers has meant that despite heavy lobbying by the pharmaceutical interests promoting BST, the European Union has agreed a ban on it until the year 2000.

INTENSIVE DAIRY FARMING AND THE ENVIRONMENT

The modern intensive dairy farm specialises in milk production only, not mixed activities such as growing crops or rearing animals for meat. The beauty of the traditional mixed farm, in theory anyway, is that it can recycle all the waste it produces. Waste from the dairy can be used as fertiliser, it can grow its own winter feed for milkers and so on.

These days British milk production is dominated by a relatively small number of dairy-only farms, which are reliant on buying in food as concentrates. The high-yielding cows fed on their high-protein diet produce vast amounts of waste which cannot be recycled within the farm.

Dairy farms have been identified as the single biggest source of water pollution in the UK. This is from not only the slurry generated by the cows but also the widespread use of silage (fermented grass) as a winter food. Silage 'run-off' (the seeping out of liquid) is thought to be 200 times more polluting than untreated human sewage. One intensive dairy farm can have the same impact as a small town on water pollution levels. This is one of the reasons why many rural rivers are now showing urban levels of pollution.

MILK – A SENSITIVE INDICATOR OF POLLUTION

Cow's milk, like human breast milk, is a sensitive indicator of environmental pollution. Cows grazing in polluted areas will pick up pollutants and pass them on in their milk (and meat). Dioxins – toxic by-products of various chemical manufacturing processes – turn up frequently in milk. These are found in great concentrations in areas of industrial activity, such as waste incinerators, chlorine bleaching and pulp industries, chemical reprocessing plants and so on. They cause cancer and reproductive and birth defects amongst other things. Dioxins concentrate in body fat, and therefore the fat in milk. Drinking skimmed milk lowers exposure (but also affects the taste of milk). Concentrations of other toxic chemicals such as lindane and DDT are regularly found in milk, but usually at levels the government says are safe. Whether there is any such 'safe' level is debatable. Little research has been carried out into the cumulative cocktail effect of these pollutants. Buying organic milk will reduce your exposure to such toxins.

ORGANIC MILK

Organic milk is a positive alternative to milk from intensive dairy herds. Herd numbers are generally kept low. The cows graze on organic pasture that has not been treated with pesticides or fertilisers, which means that significantly fewer, if any, residues are passed on in their milk. The good health of the cows is maintained by high standards of husbandry and welfare, including natural feeding. Organic farms are encouraged to grow most of what they feed their cows, so most organic dairy farms are mixed farms.

As well as aiming to be self-sufficient in feed, there is also an emphasis on maintaining rich, varied pasture full of desirable grasses, legumes, plants and herbs, which are full of naturally occurring nutrients. (Many fields on which conventional dairy cows graze are simply sown with one or two grasses, which are encouraged to grow because of the generous use of nitrogenous fertilisers and selective weed killers.)

The use of pelleted concentrates is discouraged; when they are used, strict criteria apply, and most of them must be organic. Animal protein is banned. The diet must be 80 per cent organic, the rest from permitted natural sources. At least 60 per cent of the dry matter must come from forage, a measure which helps prevent metabolic disorders. The use of preventative antibiotics and other medicines is not allowed. Organic dairy cows cannot be kept indoors or tethered permanently, and adequate bedding must always be provided for their comfort. Because they are fed a natural diet they do not produce the huge milk yield expected of the intensively farmed dairy cow, and therefore are under less strain. Organic calves stay with their mothers for much longer than calves in conventional systems.

HOW COW'S MILK IS ALTERED BEFORE YOU DRINK IT

Farmers either sell their milk to large dairies or bottle and carton it themselves to sell to the public. In the first case, the milk is picked up by a huge tanker, which travels round numerous farms in the area, and taken to a central dairy for treatment. The milk can be stored for up to 12 hours at the dairy and is then called 'accommodation milk'. The bigger the dairy, the more likely there is to be a mix of milks from different sources, known as 'reload milk'. Farms with their own dairy usually treat only their own milk. As a general rule, milk from small on-farm dairies is likely to be of the highest standard, since it is sold direct to the public. Its good reputation lies exclusively in that farm's output. You can go and see the farm if you want, and find out whether it lies next to a chemical reprocessing plant (see page 154) or amongst green rolling hills. Milk from on-farm dairies will not have travelled around in a tanker, will be bottled quickly and passed through fewer pipes and factory lines. Some supermarket milk will be bought direct from farms with specially selected herds. This is usually indicated on the label.

All dairies, on-farm or off, have to take bacterial counts from each batch of milk to ensure that it does not rise above an agreed level. Premiums are paid to farmers according to the cleanliness of the milk. In order to kill off any pathogenic bacteria which could be harmful to health, and to give the milk a longer shelf life, the raw milk is **pasteurised**.

Pasteurisation was introduced earlier this century as a measure to prevent the spread of tuberculosis. In England and Wales the sale of raw milk is still allowed, while in Scotland and Ireland it is illegal.

Pasteurisation provokes mixed opinions. The majority view is that it is an essential, if minimum, guarantee of food safety. Advocates of raw milk, on the other hand, see pasteurised milk as a denatured food – the process also kills off certain vitamins, beneficial bacteria and volatile aromas which give the milk much of its flavour. They argue that pasteurisation is often used as a prop by farmers whose milk is not clean enough to start with, while raw milk producers are extra-meticulous in their hygiene standards.

If you want to buy unpasteurised (green top) milk, make sure it is from an accredited herd with tuberculosis-free status.

In the UK 99 per cent of milk sold for drinking is pasteurised. In addition, most of it is **homogenised**, a process that distributes the fat particles more finely throughout the milk and improves its keeping qualities. Some milk sold in bottles from on-farm dairies is not homogenised, which means that the fat will rise to the top – 'the top of the milk'. Increasingly, milk in glass jars from dairies is homogenised, and milk sold in cartons always is. Homogenisation does not have to be declared on the label so most cartons don't specify it, but bottled homogenised milk from dairies usually has a different cap. The colour codes for milk bottle tops are:

- silver – full-fat milk that has not been homogenised
- red – homogenised full-fat milk
- silver with red stripe – semi-skimmed milk
- silver with blue stripe – skimmed milk
- green – unpasteurised milk
- gold – milk from higher-fat breeds, such as Jersey and Guernsey

Ordinary drinking milk can be further treated. It can be **skimmed**, so that a proportion of fat is removed (see page 158). It can be **vitaminised** – synthetic vitamins and minerals are added to compensate for those destroyed by pasteurisation. This gives it a healthy aura but it only replaces the goodness that would have been there in the first place. And it can be **ultra heat-treated** (known as UHT) or **sterilised**, an extreme form of pasteurisation. Both these treatments mean that the milk can be stored unrefrigerated for some months.

All of these interventions alter the natural character of the milk and affect its flavour to a greater or lesser extent. Homogenisation makes quite a difference to the texture and mouth-feel. Removing fat affects flavour for the worse (see below). Heat treatment leaves a perceptible 'cooked' taste and depletes vitamins, either straight away, or while the milk is in storage.

Powdered milk is simply milk (usually low fat) that has had its water evaporated away. **Evaporated** milk is sterilised milk that has been concentrated and its water content reduced. **Condensed** milk is reduced and usually sweetened. Even when unsweetened, the lactose (natural sugar) in the milk caramelises slightly with heating, giving it its characteristic flavour. Obviously, neither condensed nor evaporated milk is consumed as ordinary drinking milk.

THE FAT IN MILK

Milk is not a high-fat food but you might be forgiven for thinking that it was. More than half the milk we drink has been fat-reduced. Many consumers buy it because they think it will make an important contribution to lowering their total fat intake. In fact, **full-fat milk** contains no more than 3–5 per cent fat, depending on the breed of cow. **Semi-skimmed milk** contains 1.5–1.8 per cent fat and **skimmed milk** contains less than 0.3 per cent. So you would have to drink an awful lot of milk before a change to lower-fat milks made any great impact on your fat intake, or even approximated to the hidden fat in a couple of digestive biscuits!

Any fat-reduction benefit from a change to lower-fat milk is at the expense of flavour. The fatty acids in milk are mainly what gives it its taste, along with certain enzymes and volatile aromas. These enzymes and aromas are killed off by pasteurisation, so in pasteurised milk the last hope for flavour comes in the form of the fatty acids. Skim these off and you are left with something that tastes thin and watery.

MILK – THE BEST-TASTING BREEDS

Most of the milk we drink comes from **Friesian** or **Holstein** cows, or a cross between the two. These large cows have become increasingly popular with farmers, since they produce more milk than any other type. Their calves are strong for a dairy breed, and can often be sold for beef production. Friesian–Holstein milk has an average 3.9 per cent fat.

More traditional dairy breeds in the UK are smaller, neater cows and these are famous for the taste of their milk – the **Ayrshire, Jersey** and **Guernsey**. This reputation for flavour lies in the higher fat content of their milk. Ayrshire milk has about 4.1 per cent, Jersey 5.4 per cent and Guernsey 4.7 per cent. In addition, Ayrshire milk has a very good distribution of small fat globules, which is thought to make it specially good for cheese-making. Jersey milk has a higher proportion of desirable solids that are not fat, and therefore attracts a premium price.

Traditional breeds have been edged out to a certain extent by the high-yielding Friesian and Holstein because of the unfashionably higher fat content of their milk and the fact that their calves are not well-adapted to beef production. These traditional milks have nevertheless maintained a following amongst taste-led consumers. More retailers are including them in their range and so they are nearly always available. This type of milk usually sells in supermarkets as 'breakfast milk'.

Cream and crème fraîche

Cream is the fat that comes to the surface of milk before any homogenisation has taken place. It is simply skimmed off the milk, or alternatively spun in a mechanical separator. As with milk, cream reflects the breed of cow and their diet. Channel Island breeds produce richer cream which is higher in fat. Different pastures produce cream with distinctive flavours. All the factors affecting quality in milk also affect cream.

Otherwise, cream is usually sold on the basis of its fat content: **double cream** (48 per cent), **whipping cream** (35 per cent), **single cream** (18 per cent), **half cream**, which is half cream half milk (12 per cent). Apart from counting calories, all this tells you is the cream's ability to whip. The higher the fat, the stiffer it will be. Below 35 per cent it will not whip. The exception to the rule is French-style **crème fraîche épaisse**. This is cream that has been thickened either by natural bacteria which occur in unpasteurised milk or by the more modern method of treating pasteurised cream with a lactic culture, which thickens and sets the milk. This also gives it a pleasantly sour flavour. Crème fraîche is a fairly high-fat cream, with a fat content between 35 and 40 per cent. However, as it is set and thick it is a slightly healthier (lower-fat) alternative to double cream because it gives the feeling of richness and thickness without quite so many calories.

These days there are lots of 'low-fat' versions of crème fraîche with varying fat contents. Even in its high-fat form, it is no good for whipping. In France whipped cream is made from a thinner type of crème fraîche called *liquide* or *fluide*, which is not sold in the UK. When buying *crème fraîche épaisse*, check the label for undesirable additives such as starch, other thickeners and preservatives. These are sometimes included in the low-fat British versions and they spoil the texture, giving the cream an ersatz thickness.

British **soured cream** is relatively low-fat cream (20 per cent) that has been slightly thickened by the use of lactic cultures.

Smetana (10 per cent) is a lower-fat alternative to soured cream, made from soured cream and skimmed milk. **Extra-thick cream** is made by mechanically breaking up the fat in the cream into smaller pieces, which has the effect of thickening it.

Some French creams, such as Isigny Sainte-Mère, are protected by **AOC** status (Appellation d'Origine Contrôlée), because their milk is thought to be so special. There is no equivalent in the UK.

Clotted cream, like crème fraîche, is destined for spooning, not whipping. The cream is heated so that it sets (hence the 'cooked' flavour) and then skimmed off. It contains 55 per cent fat.

Cream substitutes are available but these are usually various combinations of buttermilk, vegetable oils, emulsifiers and additives that have no place in wholesome, high-quality food. They may be lower fat but, like margarine (see page 241) they taste artificial, have none of the good flavour of natural dairy produce, and are a totally synthetic food. If you are worried about the fat in cream, either choose the lower-fat varieties such as single cream, smetana and soured cream, eat it in smaller quantities, or choose a natural lower-fat substitute such as fromage frais or a good yogurt.

Butter and buttermilk

Butter is made by churning cream. The butter is the solid mass of fat (around 80 per cent) produced by this process and **buttermilk** is the liquid whey that remains. This latter product is ideal for baking, in recipes such as Irish soda bread, because the acids in it act with bicarbonate of soda and encourage the bread to rise without causing that slightly sherbety baking soda aftertaste. Buttermilk is most commonly made now by adding cultures to skimmed milk.

Salted butter can have up to 2 per cent salt added. **Unsalted butter** is also known in the USA as sweet butter. Salt content is no reflection of quality and the choice of unsalted or salted butter is a matter of preference. There are some really excellent salted butters, and some really horrible ones. The same applies to unsalted.

Concentrated butter is just clarified butter. The protein and salts in the butter are removed by heating, leaving a clearer mass which will not burn when cooked. This type of butter can be useful in certain recipes – when frying, for example – but cannot automatically be substituted for butter without other adjustments. 'Intervention' milk from the European milk lake is the standard source of this product. **Ghee**, used in Indian cooking, is another type of clarified butter, where the milk solids and sugar have been caramelised and removed. It is good for cooking but you can substitute vegetable oil.

All the quality factors affecting milk also affect butter. Butter labelling is spectacularly uninformative as a rule. The basic milk can have come from several sources. It can be what is known as 'accommodation' or 'reload' milk (see page 156) or it can be frozen milk. Quite a lot of butter is made from 'intervention' milk. You can spot this by the label, which says 'product of several countries'. A few small on-farm dairies still make their own butter. This is worth buying because the milk used is likely to be much fresher.

Some **French butters** are protected by AOC (Appellation d'Origine Contrôlée) status, such as **Charentes-Poitou, Isigny Sainte-Mère** and **Deux Sèvres**. The milk must come from a strict geographical area and must conform to tight quality controls. This butter is usually only available in specialist shops and prestige supermarket branches.

There is a clear difference in style between British, Irish and former Commonwealth butters, and imported butters – usually French and Danish. The first are generally made with cream which, though it may have been aged for a couple of days, has had no lactic cultures added to ripen or slightly ferment the milk. This produces butter with a neutral flavour. French butters, on the other hand, are made with milk that has been treated with lactic cultures, which gives the butter much more flavour – a slightly sharp edge and a faintly nutty-cheesy quality. Danish butter uses lactic cultures, too, but the style is less pronounced than the French ones.

Freshly churned butter is just a meaningless marketing term, like 'farm-fresh' and has no legal definition. **Easy-spread butters** are regular butters that have either been chilled and then whipped with air or have had the fat removed, the hard fat separated out and the soft fat put back in. The product has been more heavily processed but it is easier to spread.

Yogurt, fromage frais . . . and other white things in pots

There is a phenomenal number of white things in pots these days and making a good choice is not always easy.

Yogurt is milk, either whole or skimmed, that has been heated and soured by the addition of lactic cultures, *Lactobacillus bulgaricus* and *Streptococcus thermophilus*. Cow's, sheep's and goat's milk can all be used, though cow's milk is the most common. **Set yogurt** has had the culture added to it in the pot. Regular or **runny yogurt** has it added before it goes into pots. **Greek-style yogurt** (which can be either cow's or sheep's milk) is similar to ordinary yogurt but uses a different strain of lactic culture. Strictly speaking, these should be called **fermented milks** not yogurt. **Strained yogurt** has had some of its whey removed, making it richer and thicker.

Yogurts made with the lactic cultures *Lactobacillus acidophilus* and *bifidus* are sold on the basis that these bacteria stimulate the immune system and help balance the bacteria in your gut. Don't put too much faith in these claims. There is little proof that modern commercial **'live' yogurts** can do that job. It is doubtful whether they contain enough of these bacteria to have a beneficial effect or whether they remain live for long enough when on our shelves.

Fromage frais and **quark** are fresh cheeses made by curdling milk with enzymes, which means they do not have any of the notional benefits associated with the lactic cultures in yogurt. They are usually beaten first to make them smooth.

All of these products in their virgin form are healthy, natural, wholesome, and as good as the milk from which they were produced, as well as being good sources of calcium and protein. There is very little to be gained in fat-reduction terms by favouring special low-fat versions and everything to be lost in flavour. Low-fat yogurts taste like slightly thickened white water, and the very lowest grades of fromage frais and quark are fairly unpleasant. Like milk (see page 158), it is the fatty acids that give these products their flavour.

Once you move out of the sphere of relatively simple and natural yogurt and fromage frais, you enter the territory of the pudding. The healthy image of these flavoured desserts exploited by manufacturers to sell very heavily processed products with large numbers of additives. This is particularly the case with 'low-fat' products, which are fairly unpalatable in their basic form. So when you buy this type of product, remember that it should be a fairly simple one, with a very short ingredients listing. The longer the list, the more adulterated, the more processed and the less healthy it will be.

The basic **set fruit yogurts** without bits, and **flavoured fromage frais**, contain added sugar or low-calorie sweeteners such as aspartame. Though lower calorie than sucrose or white sugar, such sweeteners usually have a much more intensely sweet and, some find, very chemical flavour. More disguised sugar is often added in the form of very sweet juices, such as apple or mango.

Yogurts and fromage frais are usually flavoured with either synthetic or 'nature-identical' fruit flavours. The former have to be declared on the label as 'flavouring'. Most **fruit yogurts** with bits in are made with a commercial fruit base containing a preservative to make it last. Colourings from natural sources, but not natural to this category of product, are commonly added. Fromage frais and quark are often made with skimmed milk (sounds healthier) but have cream added. This obviously nullifies any low-fat advantage. Thickeners and emulsifiers, such as gelatine, modified starch, carob and guar gum, pectin and carrageen, are frequently used to give a good 'mouth-feel'. Yet all of them are unnecessary and, in certain cases, suspect additives which we would be better off without. To con you into thinking that this is all very good for you, some fashionable lactic cultures and extra vitamins are often added.

Worst of all are milk-based **flans, mousses and cream desserts**, which are invariably extremely sweet, full of vegetable fat and contain a long list of other dubious additives. Some quality products do exist but you need to check the ingredients label. They should contain only the sort of ingredients you would use at home, such as cream, fruit and sugar.

Ice cream and frozen yogurt

In its finest and simplest form, ice cream is simply a good egg custard – milk, cream, egg, sugar, natural vanilla – that has been churned and frozen. These days there is a great gulf in the ice cream market. High-quality or 'premium' ice creams contain only variations on these base ingredients, with other additions such as fruit purée and nuts. They are expensive because they are made with good-quality natural ingredients and only a small amount of air is whipped into them – just enough to let you get the spoon in.

Then there are the considerably cheaper ice creams (just read the label to tell them apart) which are essentially foul combinations of skimmed milk or reconstituted milk powders, loads of sugar and sweeteners, hardened vegetable fats, emulsifiers, colourings, flavourings, acidity regulators and other totally artificial processing aids, all whipped up with voluminous quantities of air. When the exact composition of dairy ingredients drops below a certain level, such products have to be called 'non-dairy ice cream' or 'frozen dessert'. Beware! You have been warned…

Frozen yogurt is a lower-fat alternative to proper ice cream. As with ice cream, upmarket versions are just what they seem, a natural product that has been frozen. Downmarket versions suffer from all the adulterations associated with yogurt (see page 163), with some air whipped in for good measure.

Selecting cheese

There is a phenomenal variety of cheese on sale these days but it is not always obvious which are the good ones. Generic names such as Parmesan, Cheddar and Camembert have become entirely meaningless. They are used indiscriminately to describe a *type* of cheese but tell you absolutely nothing about the *quality* of a specific version in that category.

Like salami, cheeses throughout Europe have suffered from modern technology. Many on sale now are second-rate factory copies of great traditional cheeses. Some countries have made an industry out of producing compromised commercial versions of other countries' classic cheeses. It is a crazy world where German 'Brie' and Danish 'feta' are as commonplace as the real thing, and may even have supplanted it.

Though a few detailed protection schemes operate for a limited number of foreign cheeses, offering a guarantee for the vigilant, most people remain baffled. The ultimate irony is that there is an increasing number of high-quality cheeses on offer, both traditional and modern. The problem is distinguishing them – an effort which pays off in the end. When you know how to buy well, cheese transforms itself from a boring weekly staple into one of life's great pleasures.

THE IMPORTANCE OF THE MILK

At its simplest, cheese is just curdled or soured milk. The single most important factor in cheesemaking therefore is the quality of the milk. Just as with meat, the flavour and goodness of milk varies according to the way the animals are kept and, most importantly, what they eat. A herd of dairy cows out chewing the cud in lush, natural pastures full of clover and other wild grasses will produce infinitely superior milk to those who are fed indoors on a large proportion of bought-in feed and sent out occasionally to graze on fields next to the municipal rubbish dump!

In Normandy you will see black and white cows with distinctive face markings which make them look as if they are wearing sunglasses. Their milk has a singular flavour which is attributed to the slight saltiness of their pastures, which are never far from the sea. Animals feeding on organic pastures obtain much of their goodness from naturally occurring nutrients in the pasture, not chemical inputs, and that will influence the flavour. Different breeds of animals produce particular types of milk, too. Jersey or Guernsey cows, for example, produce particularly rich and unctuous cheese because of the relatively high fat content of their milk (see page 159).

Since the quality of the milk is fundamental to the quality of the cheese, it is essential that the source is protected and carefully controlled. The best traditional foreign cheeses have created a legal protection for their milk. The top Parmesan, parmigiano reggiano (see page 178), can only be made from the milk of cows from a very specific geographical area subject to tight controls. The same applies to the sheep's milk used in Roquefort. None of the classic British cheeses have this type of protection except Stilton.

The best versions of the traditional British cheeses, and the impressive modern ones, try to control the quality by other means. They are what is known as 'on-farm cheeses', where the same company or individual controls both the milk production and the cheesemaking. Cheeses made from milk that is bought in are very different because the cheesemaker does not have total control over production. At worst, this leads to the situation found in the handful of highly automated industrial creameries that dominate mass production. Milk is pooled from a variety of different sources, picked up by a giant tanker which travels around a geographical area over a number of days. In this system, milk is often stored refrigerated for days at a time before being made into cheese. Although there is no evidence to suggest that this milk is not wholesome in microbiological terms – cell counts for bacteria are taken at all farms and so on – farmers selling into a pool are in the business of producing a standard commodity, with no particular motivation to see that the milk is first class. Produce it, sell it – a simple economic transaction.

Small-scale cheesemakers who have to buy in milk tend to be choosier about its quality, usually sticking to a known farm, although they do not have total control over its production. However, they are very much at the whim of market forces, especially fluctuations in milk prices. This instability can put them out of business.

THE SKILLS OF THE CHEESEMAKER

Even the best milk can be ruined if cheesemakers do not know what they are doing. Cheesemaking is an art. In very simple cheeses, such as fresh goat's cheese, cottage and cream cheese, the milk is soured by adding a lactic acid starter, allowed to drain and then sold within a matter of days.

For more complex cheeses, which will be matured and aged, the milk is then curdled or coagulated with rennet, either animal-derived or vegetarian (see page 182). The curds are cut and formed, slightly 'cooked' if it is a firm cheese, formed into moulds, then dry-salted or dipped in brine. In blue cheeses, thin needles are introduced which allows air to penetrate and encourages the characteristic blue veins to develop.

Once the cheeses are taken from their moulds the next stage is maturing, anything from a matter of weeks to years according to the type of cheese. Some are simply turned at regular intervals and dried out progressively. Others are washed in alcohols and other liquids to encourage them to develop a special taste and aroma, or stored in special environments which promote the formation of a white bloomy rind or a crumbly crust. Traditional, British cheeses are wrapped in cloth to allow them to breathe as they mature.

Proper 'farmhouse' or hand-made cheese production calls for skilled and highly experienced craftspeople who have to make key judgements on each batch of milk. Much depends on how long the curd is left with the whey, the size of the curd, and the level of acidity that is allowed to develop. All this influences the character of the cheese and the speed at which it will mature, while seasonal variations in the milk can alter the way that it handles. Such decisions require great experience.

In large-scale industrial cheesemaking, the production process is entirely automated – a push-button, computer-controlled exercise whose goal it is to push more product through the system quickly in order to make a swift return on investment. Most factory cheeses are made to different recipes from their genuine farmhouse equivalents. The maturing process is usually quite different too. In factory form, the famous English territorials – Cheddar, Cheshire, Lancashire, Wensleydale, Caerphilly and so on – are effectively matured in plastic bags, which inhibit the development of individual character. This produces bland and characterless cheese which is sold far too young.

Even more pathetic are the attempts of the large creameries to diversify when criticised for being boring. This has spawned a whole list of pseudo-cheeses sold as 'speciality' cheeses when they are in fact only the same boring product with dubious additives – herbs and meat flavourings, colourings, emulsifiers – formed with contrasting lines, funny faces and more of that ilk.

FIRST FIND YOUR SOURCE

Cheese retailing is not one of our national strengths. Traditionally, grocers bought a couple of cheeses from their nearest supplier, usually local cheeses, faithful to their farmhouse roots. In the 1970s and 1980s, delicatessens took on the role. They sold the growing number of ubiquitous industrial versions of these traditional cheeses and a number of misunderstood foreign imports that were generally of mediocre factory standard.

British supermarkets, in contrast to European ones, have always been spectacularly unimpressive in the cheese they stock. They are quite good at handling certain kinds of cheese. If it needs chilling – feta, ricotta and so on – supermarket cold chains can be much more effective at delivering the cheese in good condition.

But, as always, they will offer you the most standardised version of that product. Supermarket mozzarella or ricotta, for example, can never compare with the more authentic brands you'll find in good Italian food shops. Only a few decent foreign cheeses manage to penetrate the supermarket wall of blandness. They tend to come in a pretty box, or already wrapped by the producer, so they can be sold individually. As for traditional favourites, supermarket ranges are still overwhelmingly dependent on factory cheeses, sold in cuts off a block and uninformatively labelled by country (English, Scottish, Irish) and unspecified age (mild, mature, extra mature).

Descriptions such as these are not measured to any set of objective standards. One factory's 'extra mature' often tastes milder than another's 'mature'. The maturity might come from fairly traditional ageing over months or simply because more acid has been allowed to develop in the cheese at the beginning, giving it a stronger flavour.

On the delicatessen counter, the lack of knowledge about both cheese and cheese retailing means that any cheese with style or character is in the minority, and badly misunderstood. The chances are it won't sell so it will be 'de-listed', or dropped. In supermarkets, the information that consumers really need about cheese is hardly ever on the label. Is it a factory cheese or a genuine farmhouse product? What age is it? Is it ready to eat? Is the milk drawn from one named farm or several in a region? The truth is that if you want answers to these questions, you will have to find a specialist cheese shop whose staff are informed enough to fill in some of the missing information.

RECOGNISING A GOOD CHEESE SHOP

Because there has been a renaissance in small-scale British cheese-making, many more specialist retailers with expertise and knowledge in the field (and much better cheese) are springing up. Supermarkets have been unable to mount any serious threat to small, specialist cheese shops offering distinctive cheeses with some style and character. Very few genuine farmhouse cheese-makers can supply the volume of cheese that the big chains demand to make it worth their while. In this sector of food retailing the small shop is flourishing. Most major centres of population have such an outlet, and it is worth making it your first port of call.

There are two aspects to making a good purchase. The first is that the cheese should be in good condition. That means that you are being given a good example of its type. The second is the range on offer. Retailers who look after their cheeses are more likely to take care in their selection, too.

- The wrappings on the cheeses should be clean, tight and shiny, looking as though they are changed daily – no tatty bits of greasy clingfilm. The very best specialist cheese shops control the temperature with air-conditioning so the cheeses are kept cold and damp. Such shops do not always wrap their cheeses and that is perfectly acceptable.
- The labels or cards on the cheese should be clean and clearly written, not smudged and grubby.
- The cheese cabinet or counter should look nice and clean, and not cramped – this encourages neglect!
- There should be a small, well-selected range of cheese which is obviously turning over fast. The choice should be fairly limited in all but a handful of really top specialist shops, who are geared up to cope with a larger range.

As well as looking after the cheese, the retailers need to be capable of selling it. So:

- Give your business to shops where the staff seem keen on their subject and like to talk about it.
- Only buy cheese from shops that encourage you to taste, rather than giving you some grudgingly when asked.

From there on it, there are a number of indicators that a cheese will be good. The more of these you can put a tick against, the better.

- **Price (unfortunately)**: If you want a cheese with some individuality and style, don't drop below £3 a pound.

- **Descriptions:** Unless your retailer is downright fraudulent, labels such as 'farmhouse', 'on-farm', 'hand-made' and 'artisanal' are a good indicator of quality.
- **Labels**: Good signs include marks such as French AOC (Appellation d'Origine Contrôllée) and Italian DT or DO (Denominazione Tipica, Denominazione d'Origine), Spanish DO (Denominacion d'Origen), trade consortium (*conzorzio*) logos, '*fermier*', meaning farmhouse, on French cheeses, '*artisanale*', meaning hand-made, on Italian cheeses, or European Union 'Certificate of Specific Character' status. Specially good imported cheeses often have a quality mark as described, *plus* the name of the person who has matured and/or produced them (for example, Brie de Meaux *Rouzaire*, Gorgonzola Dolce *Peck*). This means that these are thought to be exceptionally good in their class and sell on their name.
- **Raw milk**: The finest cheeses are made with raw (unpasteurised) milk (see page 180). They tend to have much more character and flavour.
- **Natural coverings**: Cloth-wrapped hard cheeses have usually been matured in a traditional manner which enables them to breathe. Waxed rind cheeses and those wrapped in plastic, or those without a natural rind, have not.
- **No pseudo-cheeses**: A decent cheese retailer would not be seen dead with a block of pizza-, ham-, apricot- or chutney-flavoured cheese. These are marketing gimmicks invented to add value to boring factory cheese – both British and imported. While certain herbs and seasonings are legitimate ingredients in a small number of traditional cheeses (such as the rosemary, juniper and savory on Corsican Brin d'Amour, or the ash on French goat's cheeses), these are easy to tell apart from the silly newcomers.

Be careful about smoked cheeses. Some are naturally smoked, others are simply dipped in an artificial flavouring called liquid smoke (see page 136), which is revolting.

BIG CHEESE

On the whole, the bigger the cheese of its type, the better. When you buy a cheese such as a Cheddar or Stilton, a slice from a large wheel tends to taste much better than a wedge from a small truckle. However attractive truckles and other mini versions may appear, they do not have the same eating qualities as a big cheese. This is because there is more crust or rind in relation to the centre, and also because smaller cheeses dry out more quickly.

This does not apply to all cheeses. Some cheeses, such as French goat's cheeses, are traditionally made small and destined to be sold individually. These fresher kinds of cheeses would not hold together easily if they were any bigger.

Watch out for 'baby' versions of larger cheese. Many of these have literally been dreamed up over the last decade for the growing cheeseboard market. Usually the marketing is better than the flavour.

THE CHARACTERISTICS OF DIFFERENT MILKS AND THEIR CHEESEMAKING POTENTIAL

The animal with the most prolific milk supply is the cow, which is why the majority of cheeses come from this source. **Cow's milk** is quite neutral in flavour compared to sheep's or goat's milk because it contains fewer of the fatty acids that give milk its flavour. Cow's milk can, however, taste subtly different, depending on pasture. It is used fresh in cheeses like Greek feta, Italian mascarpone, French fromage frais and British cottage cheese. Made into hard cheese, it comes in the form of the classic English territorials (Cheddar, Cheshire and so on). When the curd is slightly cooked, you get firm, very smooth cheeses such as French

Gruyère and Comté, or Swiss Emmenthal, which are highly prized for their melting abilities.

When it is youthful, cow's milk cheese is pleasant but quite bland. Depth of flavour comes with ageing. Firm cheeses of the Cheddar type develop acidity, which gives them their mature flavour. Aged in the Italian way, cow's milk can make extremely hard, granular cheeses of tremendous character, such as parmigiano reggiano (see page 178). Softer, younger cow's milk cheeses with pronounced flavours include the white 'bloomy rind' cheeses such as Brie de Melun and Brie de Meaux, and orangey-coloured 'washed-rind' cheeses such as French Reblochon, or Irish Gubbeen. This type of maturation produces cheeses that, although they have pungent aromas, are often quite mild in taste. The French make exceptionally rich and buttery *triple crème* cheeses such as the traditional Explorateur and the modern Pavé d'Affinois.

Sheep's milk has much more character from day one, with a heavier flavour and an aroma more like evaporated milk. Very little sheep's milk cheese is made to be eaten fresh, such as Corsican Brousse. Most is semi-hard, such as Sardinian pecorino, Spanish Manchego, Basque Brébis and English Beenleigh Blue. Spanish and Italian sheep's milk cheeses are often aged. They dry out, form a very tough rind, rather like Parmesan, and have a very concentrated rich flavour.

Goat's milk has a fresh, slightly sharp, chalky flavour which lends itself especially to fresh cheeses destined for short maturation. French classics include the variously shaped (log, pyramid, square, thimble) cheeses such as St Maure, crottin de Chavignol and Valençay. Fresh English goat's cheese like Innes and Perroche are in the same style. Aged goat's cheeses can be crumbly, intense and wonderful but some others can be too concentrated in flavour and almost inedible.

Buffalo's milk is the proper ingredient for the finest Italian mozzarella, provolone and scamorza. It has a higher fat content than either cow's, sheep's or goat's milk, which accounts, in part, for its deliciousness. It is hard to come by, so cow's milk is often substituted but this does not have the rich, creamy, yielding depths of the real thing.

JUDGING CHEESES

Use your nose

All cheese, even hard cheese, should have an attractive smell that makes you want to eat it. Anything odourless is probably immature, sterile and characterless. Strong smells are fine and, indeed, essential in washed and bloomy-rind cheeses, such as Camembert or Pont l'Eveque. Cheese that smells of ammonia or has a rancid odour is unacceptable. If it has a sweaty smell it may be all right but it needs to be left unwrapped for a while.

Use your eyes

Hard cheese should look smooth. There should not normally be any blue mould in non-blue cheeses, although in certain very mature farmhouse cheeses a small amount is considered acceptable by connoisseurs and not seen as a fault, rather as a sign that it has been well aged. Soft cheeses with washed or bloomy rinds should fill their skins or crusts well, and neither be splitting open or sunken down and withered looking (overripe). Fresh cheeses such as goat's cheese crottins should look even coloured and free of mould or bloom. Matured goat's and sheep's milk cheeses can look like something from a mummy's tomb but still taste fantastic.

Use your tastebuds

All good cheese, even hard cheese, melts on the roof of your mouth. More complex cheeses should have a greater length of flavour. If it sticks to the roof of your mouth, is unyielding, has no flavour, tastes of aluminium foil (blue cheese), or reminds you of soap – don't eat it! Very fresh cheeses such as ricotta or fromage frais should never have a sherbety, slightly fizzy quality – if they do, they are too old. Anything that tastes of mould or reminds you of dirty dishcloths is irretrievably flawed.

Use your head

Taste your way around the possibilities in a category. Take blues, for example. Try a factory Danablu or Bresse bleu against Stilton and Gorgonzola (all cow's milk cheeses). Compare a Roquefort and a Bleu d'Auvergne (sheep's milk versus cow's milk). Try two different types of Roquefort against each other . . . and so on. Paying attention to what you buy will inform your next purchase.

THE GEOGRAPHY OF GOOD CHEESE

When buying cheese you are allowed to have national prejudices! Some countries are good at cheese, others are, well, less so. Here's a whistle-stop tour.

England produces a huge range of interesting hand-made cheeses, both traditional and modern. Great classics include **Appleby's Cheshire, Keen's, Quicke's** and **Montgomery Cheddar, Duckett's Caerphilly** and **Colston Bassett Stilton**. Modern triumphs include **Tymsboro**', a goat's milk pyramid, sheep's milk **Beenleigh Blue** and **Spenwood**.

    Scotland used to be famous for its **Dunlop**, a variation on Cheddar. Most traditional Dunlop has now disappeared but new Scottish cheeses of note include **Bonchester** (Camembert-style), **Lanark Blue** and **Isle of Mull Cheddar**.

    Wales has surprisingly little cheese but much of what it does produce is organic. The excellence of organic **Llangloffan**, similar to good Cheshire, shows that there is tremendous potential.

    Ireland is responsible for a lot of factory Cheddar but **Carbury Creamery** still produces some good stuff. The country also produces lots of really fine hand-made cheeses, such as **Coolea, Gabriel, Desmond** (Gruyère-style), **Milleens** (washed rind) and **Durrus**, an excellent semi-hard cheese.

France continues to protect its cheeses, both old and new, offering a stunning portfolio. Essential tasting includes a good **Roquefort** such as Carles or Papillon, **Brie de Meaux, Melun** or **Nangis**, unpasteurised **Comté** (what Gruyère should be like but rarely is), the Basque **Brébis**, the **goat's cheeses** of the Ile de France and Loire, and the deliciously pongy washed-rind cheeses like **Pont l'Eveque**.

Spain distinguishes itself by producing no bad cheese. Unfortunately, it eats what it makes and very little is exported. Even factory versions of **Manchego** and **Roncal**, for example, are more than palatable, while the farmhouse versions are extremely impressive. Cow's milk **Mahon** and sheep's milk **Idiazabal** from the Basque country show the magnificence of Spanish cheesemaking.

Portugal produces mainly sheep's and goat's milk cheeses, from breeds developed specifically for cheesemaking. These are not widely available in the UK. A pity, because those such as the sheep's milk cheese **queijo da serra** show that they can be impressive.

Italy has a stunning array of cheese. The challenge is to avoid the ubiquitous industrial versions which we tend to import. **Parmigiano reggiano, Gorgonzola, buffalo's milk mozzarella** and Sardinian **pecorino** are the cornerstones.

Greece produces a limited number of cheeses. Real Greek **feta** and **halloumi** are elusive, and best bought in Greek or Cypriot shops.

And the rest? Germany's great contribution to the world of cheeses is Cambazola, its cheap and cheerless copy of Italian Gorgonzola. It is questionable whether there is any really good cheese made in Germany. If there is, it's a well-kept secret. In theory the Swiss have some good cheese. Those which impress are usually the Alpine cheeses resembling French ones. Because Switzerland is not part of the European Union, relatively few Swiss cheeses are sold in the UK. Switzerland's key export market is Germany, which doesn't do much to encourage cheeses with any style or character. Holland seems to specialise in bland rubbery cheeses of the Gouda and Edam type. Word has it that hand-made versions of these can be quite good when aged. The problem is finding them. Denmark now specialises in antiseptic factory copies of mainly blue cheese, and offers no cheeses with character. Swedish cheese is an enigma that may be solved now that Sweden has joined the European Union. A few Norwegian cheeses are sold in the UK, such as Jarlsberg. Usually, these are industrial versions and not very interesting.

PARMIGIANO REGGIANO – SO MUCH IN ONE NAME

There are a few cheeses to lay down and die for and one of them is Parmesan . . . the real thing, that is. But how do you recognise the real thing? It is called parmigiano reggiano and, unlike other Parmesan cheeses, is rigorously protected by law. Italians know what a treasure they've got.

Parmesan cheese is a member of the 'grana' family of cheeses. Real parmigiano reggiano is a moist, nutty cheese with a sweet, rich dairy aroma. Bite into it and it has an attractive crumbly, slightly gritty texture which retains little grains of salt, and a stunning intensity and complexity of flavour. The cow's milk can come only from a recognised production zone in the region of Emilia Romagna, which is protected by law. It is made to a very strict set of standards which has barely altered in the 700 years it has been in production. This stipulates traditional techniques of both making and maturing the cheese.

In Italy everyone appreciates that there is a definite hierarchy amongst Parmesans. Parmigiano reggiano is the tops, sold at two years old minimum. The very best versions of this are sold as *stravecchio* (extra old) or *stagionata* (matured) – aged for anything up to five years.

Dropping down a quality grade, there comes a whole family of grana cheeses, which all share the same granular texture. Grana padano is the best known and looks superficially like parmigiano reggiano. These are marketed by age, from 12 to 18 months. Then there are various pecorinos, which have been put through a similar process. Though grana and aged pecorino cheeses are frequently of good everyday quality, they have neither the maturity nor the pedigree of parmigiano reggiano, and never match its eating qualities. They are always cheaper, but not substantially so – even more reason for buying parmigiano reggiano.

Finally there's the grated stuff in tubs or those miserable little pre-packs which is sold as 'Parmesan'. Although it is reminiscent of sawdust and cheese-flavoured crisps, the Italian versions are at least meant to be grana cheese. It's just a bit of a mystery how anyone can make good cheese smell and taste that bad. Industrial dehydration is the obvious culprit.

Nowadays, there is no need to settle for anything less than reggiano. All self-respecting Italian stores sell it in a wedge. Most supermarkets now sell it in fingers with only a tiny part of rind on, at a considerable mark-up. However, there is a lot to be said for the good old rind. On parmigiano reggiano, it is distinctive, bearing the name of the cheese in purplish-blue dots as an indestructible guarantee against its many imposters and frauds. Other granas just have smooth rind.

UNPASTEURISED CHEESES — BOTH FLAVOURSOME AND SAFE

All other factors being equal, unpasteurised (raw) milk will produce a better cheese, with much more character, than pasteurised milk.

Pasteurisation is used as a very minimum guarantee of milk safety. By bringing the milk to a high temperature, and holding it there for a short time, any pathogenic, or harmful bacteria are killed off. However, this also kills off many harmless bacteria, plus the volatile aromas and enzymes that give the milk its special character. The process slightly alters the flavour, too, making it blander. Such differences may be imperceptible to all but the most trained palate when tasting milk, but when it comes to cheese the difference is often accentuated. Unpasteurised cheeses always have more depth of flavour and complex character than pasteurised ones.

Many people think that by eating unpasteurised cheeses they are risking food poisoning from listeria and other bugs but this is not the case. Hard cheeses such as Cheddar are highly preserved products anyway and their natural acid inhibits pathogenic bacteria. As a result, the threat of food poisoning from them is virtually non-existent.

Soft cheeses are more prone to contamination. Very young ones such as fromage frais are usually sold quickly before pathogenic bacteria can build up, and they tend to smell bad before they pose a health risk. More mature soft cheeses, or soft-ripened cheeses, such as Brie are the least safe. But in this category of cheese, there is a lot of evidence to suggest that unpasteurised is actually safer than pasteurised. This is because beneficial bacteria remain and fight against the harmful ones, thus checking their progress. Pasteurised cheeses, on the other hand, have been made semi-sterile, which means that they are a bit like a laboratory Petri dish of agar jelly – just waiting to be colonised by any nasty bugs in the vicinity.

Many observers of the dairy trade think that some farmers use pasteurisation wrongly as a guarantee that milk can be cleaned up afterwards, and thus make less effort over basic hygiene. Producers of raw milk generally demand that the total bacteria count (TCB) of undesirable bacteria is very low because they are keen to protect the integrity of the raw milk.

LOW-FAT AND 'DIET' CHEESES

Low-fat cheese is a marketing gimmick dreamed up to add value to uninteresting, characterless cheese. It is made from skimmed or semi-skimmed milk, which means that it has a lot less flavour to start with (see page 158). Some cheeses in this category have liquid vegetable oil and hardened vegetable oil added to replace the milk fat and the flavour is terrible.

The new wave of low-fat cheeses taste even poorer than their full-fat factory equivalents, which is quite a triumph, and usually sell for a totally unjustified premium. If you are worried about fat, choose a lovely full-flavoured cheese and eat less of it (as the flavour is stronger, you will need to use less in cooking) or select a traditional one that has less fat, such as single Gloucester, fromage frais or Brie. Avoid French *triple crème* cheeses, such as Pavé d'Affinois, Gratte Paille, Pierre Robert and Explorateur, and cheeses made from higher-fat Jersey and Guernsey milk.

PROCESSED CHEESE

Squirting cheeses, spreading cheeses, cheese in cubes, cheese in triangles . . . these have been processed so they can be made into these forms. A cheese of very basic quality is chopped up, melted and mulched (frequently broken down into various constituent chemical parts – casein, lactose and so on) with a motley array of additives. These include both synthetic and natural colours, various sugars, preservatives (to render the destabilised mass 'safe' and give it a long shelf life), antioxidant synergists (to bind the various elements together and give it a good 'mouth-feel') and emulsifiers (to thicken and add bulk). Enough said.

VEGETARIAN CHEESE

The customary substance used to curdle or coagulate milk for cheese is an enzyme called rennet, which is derived from the stomach of an animal, usually a calf. This is a problem for vegetarians since it is an animal product, and so more cheeses are being made with a non-animal derived coagulant.

Various plants can be used. Portuguese queijo da serra cheese is curdled with nettle juice. Cardoon (thistle) flowers, safflower seed, plants such as lady's bedstraw and certain tree saps will all have the desired effect. But these days, the most common substitute is a copy of rennin derived from the yeast mould, Mucor.

One other vegetarian alternative now being adopted by large-scale cheesemakers is a new genetically engineered copy enzyme called chymosin. This is a rather controversial substitute, since there are concerns over the lack of testing and controls on genetically altered foods. It has only been used for a few years, and is not tried and tested over time in the way that animal rennet is.

Cheeses made using chymosin are sold as vegetarian but only a few retailers indicate on the label that this means genetically altered. This is because the cheese is only made *with the aid of* genetic technology, and does not actually contain the GMO (genetically modified organism). You would think that *any* application of genetic engineering would be essential information to the consumer, but you cannot take that for granted! (See page 286.)

Bread

You have probably already formed your opinion of the state of British breadmaking. These days there is a stark contrast between the standard industrial sliced loaf which dominates the market and the new breads. These are made to traditional methods by modern enthusiasts and they are beginning to make their presence felt. No other European country has gone over to industrial bread-making in such an overwhelming way, as we all discover when we travel abroad. Yet in response to this attack on traditional skills, a new generation of specialist breadmakers has come to the fore. Good British bread – when you can find it – is as good as you can buy anywhere. However, locating good bread is increasingly becoming a geographical problem, with interesting breads available only to those who seek them out in cosmopolitan, urban areas. Out of town, industrial pap too often rules the roost.

Some consumers make do with the standard offerings because they do not know where to look for anything with more character. Others turn to baking their own. The middle ground for many people, though, is tracking down bread which is really worth getting enthusiastic about.

If you have already written off standard industrial British bread, you can easily skip the section that follows on what is known politely as 'the sliced and wrapped' loaf. If you just want positive pointers about finding good bread, move directly on to Recognising Good Bread and Finding Better Bread.

Alternatively, you might like to know how British breadmaking went so badly wrong.

How most British bread is produced

Nowadays 80 per cent of the product we are sold as 'bread' is what is known as 'sliced and wrapped'. Whether it is called white, brown, stoneground, malted, multi-grain, soft-grain or high energy is largely an irrelevance. Though the ingredient mix may vary, these are all just variations on the same theme.

These are loaves churned out on a massive industrial scale by a small number of huge bread plants. In these plants, traditional baking skills have been superseded by an entirely automated, computer-controlled process, which can produce a cooled, sliced and wrapped loaf in three and a half hours from start to finish. A typical bread plant can produce as many as 6,600 loaves an hour. All this is thanks to a fast-track bread production system known as the Chorleywood Bread Process (CBP).

The CBP, or 'no-time' process as it is sometimes also known, was developed in 1961. It was a disaster for British bread. The UK now has the lowest bread consumption of any European country – a testimony to how joyless, uniform and fundamentally unsatisfying our bread has become. Bread made by this type of process is almost non-existent in other European countries.

The CBP differs substantially from traditional craft bakery techniques. One key difference is that the traditional slow, patient kneading of the dough, followed by a long, slow fermentation period (the 'first rise', or 'bulk fermentation'), is no longer required. The CBP replaces this stage with a few minutes of intense mechanical dough development in high-speed mixers, and the quantity of yeast used is substantially increased. Using this technique, more water can be absorbed into the dough and less flour is required for each loaf. The dough rises up and reaches its desired volume much more quickly, thus dramatically shortening the breadmaking process.

Bread produced by this method has certain all too familiar characteristics. It is lightweight, pappy and insubstantial, full of air and water, with an exterior resembling soft peel or skin rather than crispy crust. The curiously unsatisfying texture of the bread is made even worse by its fundamental lack of flavour. This is largely because it has been deprived of the traditional first fermentation, which allows flavour to develop, but also because of the flour used.

FLOUR IMPROVERS AND ADDITIVES

Newly milled flour produces loaves that are smaller in volume than ones made with flour that has been aged for a few weeks, because ageing has a strengthening effect on the gluten. Traditionally, flour was left to mature for anything from three to eight weeks so that with exposure to oxygen it would become better for baking. Modern baking has developed a number of chemical 'improvers', which can be added direct to the flour. These act as oxidising agents, so the traditional maturation period can be dispensed with.

The most commonly used is **ascorbic acid** (vitamin C), which is the only improver permitted in wholemeal bread. Other improvers also bleach or whiten the flour and sterilise it at the same time, making it less prone to infestations from weevils but also removing many of its nutrients. These are chlorine dioxide, L-cysteine hydrochloride, and azodicarbonimide, which are just listed on the label as 'improvers'. **Enzyme-softening agents** may be added with the improvers to keep the bread soft and squidgy. Because these are all regarded as processing aids rather than additives, they do not need to be declared on the label. Another improver, **soya bean flour**, is used to whiten the dough and obviate the need for the first fermentation. This has to be declared.

Because white and brown flour have lost much of their nutritional goodness in the process of milling and 'improving' (see below),

by law they must have **vitamins** and certain **minerals** added –
thiamin, nicotinic acid, iron, calcium – to bring them up to an
acceptable nutritional standard. They do not contain the same
amount of **fibre** as wholemeal bread, so for bread made from a
standard white flour it is common to add fibre in the form of different parts of the wheat grain – bran, cracked wheat, wheatgerm,
oat and pea bran, sugar beet fibre and so on. These are often softened to improve the nutritional profile of the bread while retaining its characteristic soft, pappy consistency – 'soft-grain' bread.
Calcium carbonate (chalk) is frequently added to replace the
calcium lost in the modern roller-milling process, leaving over-
refined flour that has had most of its goodness milled out.
Calcium propionate can also be used to prevent mould.

A group of **emulsifiers** (E471–476) are routinely incorporated
into the dough to increase the volume of the bread and make it
softer. These also help to bind together the otherwise tricky match
of water and **vegetable fat**. This last item is incorporated to give
greater volume and slightly improved shelf life. **Vinegar** is usually
added as a mould inhibitor now that the chemicals previously used
have been banned. **Sugar** and/or **malt** are widely used to prevent the bread drying out, cut down the fermentation time and
add some flavour. **Caramel** can be added to give the crumb a
darker colour and a darker, shinier crust, while **milk powder**
gives a slightly sweet taste, disguises the basic lack of flavour in
the dough and improves shelf life.

Though none of these improvers or additives is particularly
suspect on health grounds, the question is, how can a food so
simple as bread be made so complicated? The only essential ingredients in good bread are flour, water, salt and yeast (although yeast
is dispensable – see page 194). Such additives and improvers are
unnecessary. Their presence indicates bread made from flour that
has lost most of its goodness to start with and by means of an
industrial baking technique geared to turning it out at the lowest
cost in the shortest amount of time.

If you want decent bread made from sound, simple ingredients, you will have to look beyond the wonders of the CBP sandwich loaf.

Finding better bread

It would not be hard for bread to look more appealing than the standard sliced and wrapped loaf or the flabby rolls that come out of the same industrial process. Smaller bakeries, whether local **independents, chains** or **in-store bakeries**, all produce bread that looks more promising but often disappoints. Although the CBP process is confined to the big plant bakeries, this does not mean that the intrusion of technology into traditional baking skills has stopped there.

These days, most small bakeries that still bake their bread on the premises work with the same 'improved' flour and additives used in the sliced and wrapped loaf. A vast array of equipment has been produced for bakers to allow them to make bread quicker and more profitably and cut down on anti-social working hours. Fast-acting yeasts, high-speed kneading machines, retarder machines, which bring the dough to a desired stage and then refrigerate it, electronic programmers which automatically switch it on again – these all allow bakers to stay longer in their beds at night.

Even the best supermarket instore bakeries bake bread with metered flour and water plus a little sachet containing all the additives necessary to make the dough behave. This has produced a new generation of semi-skilled bakers with only the haziest notion of traditional techniques. Such instore bakeries with even these limited skills (known as 'scratch' baking, meaning baking from scratch) are rapidly going over to ever more labour-saving techniques. The ultimate solution is the buying in of part-baked or frozen dough, known as 'bake-off'. Widely adopted by supermarkets and chain bakeries, this requires freezers and ovens but no baking skills. The dough is pre-formed at a central bakery, delivered frozen, them simply baked as required and sold as 'freshly baked' or 'baked daily'. The smell teases the money out of our wallets, and waste is cut to a minimum.

It is, of course, perfectly feasible to bake bread along traditional lines but on a commercial scale, using modern labour-saving technology. This means using decent flour (without improvers), respecting time-honoured methods (a long bulk fermentation), taking time and care in shaping the bread, and firing it in ovens capable of producing a proper crust. These craft techniques, as opposed to push-button methods, are much more likely to produce bread you can get enthusiastic about eating and which rewards your interest. However, independent craft bakers are a dying breed, and they often have only themselves to blame. Very few have seized the opportunity provided by the industrialisation of bread to specialise and make bread that is really different. Too often, they have succumbed to the temptations of prepared mixes supplied by the big millers. The result is uniformity and a general de-skilling of the trade. The most innovative small bakeries in the last 20 years have been started by people from outside the established bakery trade.

Wholefood shops do stock alternatives, but too many of these are long-life breads sold vacuum-packed. Although this may prevent mould growth, it cannot prevent the natural hardening of the starches in the loaf. The result, all too often, is like eating cardboard.

The most likely sources of good bread are the relatively small number of **craft bakeries** still baking according to traditional methods, **supermarket bread departments** (but not their instore bakeries), which sometimes stock craft breads, **specialist food shops** and **wholefood shops** which may buy in bread from high-quality, often organic, sources with relatively small outputs and limited distribution.

RECOGNISING GOOD BREAD

A certain amount can be gleaned about bread by reading the label. When it comes to a basic loaf, the shorter the list of ingredients the better. More complicated breads with additions such as olives, raisins and so on will obviously have longer ingredients lists. Nevertheless, the fewer additives and improvers the bread contains, the more wholesome it is likely to be. When making your mind up about the quality of a particular bakery outlet, judge it on its basic, most straightforward loaf, not a fancy 'speciality' bread full of extra flavours to distort your perceptions.

Designer breads are rapidly colonising our shelves and a good many of them are just the standard pappy offering baked in a new shape with some fashionable ingredients. Read the ingredients listing attentively. Sun-dried tomatoes and olive oil do not sit too happily beside milk powder and vegetable fat! And what is the point of a twenty-seed load if you cannot distinguish the flavour of any one of them?

Bread sold loose (not sliced and wrapped) does not need to have a label listing the ingredients, though they should be displayed in the shop or be available on request.

Statements of intent that actually give hard information, such as, 'We do not use improvers', 'We use organic flour', explanatory leaflets and so on are signs of bakers with a pride in their craft. But do not be taken in by twee 'Ye Olde Cottage Bakery' hype and bland assurances such as 'Traditional family bakers'. These are totally meaningless and often actively misleading.

Good bread should appeal to all the senses – sight, smell, touch, sound and taste – and really make you want to eat it. Above all, it should be satisfying. A slice of decent bread will fill you up and nourish you far more than three slices of industrial pap. Here are some ways of judging quality.

Colour of crumb

Very white bread is a sign of bleached, porous, 'improved' white flour that has had most of its goodness removed. Good white flour produces a crumb that is slightly grey, creamy or beige in colour. So-called brown or wholemeal loaves should have a fairly dark basic colour, not including any extra bits of the grain that have been added in for fibre. Pale brown bread is likely to be standard 'improved' flour with added 'bits'.

Weight

Be wary of large loaves that feel curiously light for their size. With the exception of certain light yeast breads, such as challah and milk loaves, which are meant to be that way, this is a sign of too much air and poor flour. Anything purporting to be brown or wholemeal should be reasonably heavy.

Keeping quality

Decent bread should keep reasonably well and toast satisfactorily after a few days, even lighter white breads such as bloomers and cottage loaves. The only exceptions to this are thin bread, such as the French baguette, which are best on the day they are baked. Bad bread baked in vaguely Continental shapes and styles often turns to powder and dust within hours. But a properly made baguette should still be edible sliced and toasted (if a little tough) on day two.

Bread made by traditional methods will stale eventually. Sliced and wrapped loaves may last for ages solely because enzyme-softening agents such as fungal amylase have been added with the improvers to keep the bread soft and squidgy.

Type of crust

Any loaf, of whatever style, should have a proper ratio of crust to crumb – in other words, you should be able to distinguish the two elements. Crustless loaves with peel-off skins are a tell-tale sign of bad bread. When it comes to loaves that are mainly light, white and crusty, the crust should make a satisfactory cracking noise when you press it, but it should not break into bits, a sign of over-aerated dough, too much yeast or bad flour.

Wholemeal and soda breads usually produce a hard crust which softens as it cools, so the contrast between the crust and crumb will be less marked. But you should still be able to differentiate the two when you eat it.

Much of the flavour of bread is in the crust, just like the skin of a fruit or vegetable. You can taste that in some traditionally baked batch loaves, where a side crust is deliberately avoided by placing the dough pieces so close that they touch. Such breads can have exceptionally tasty tops and bottoms.

Texture

Well-made bread, however crusty, hard or dense, should feel clean in the mouth and be easy to eat. Bread that goes gooey, gummy and then sticks to your fillings and the roof of your mouth is pappy and industrial. Heavier breads should have a decent chewy texture which tones up the gums and exercises the jaw.

Flavour

The flavour of basic breads should be nutty (like a fresh, sweet nut), satisfying and wholesome. Sourdough breads made with a leaven (see page 194) should have a slightly tangy, well-rounded flavour which you only get in well-fermented bread. Breads that taste actively sweet (unless they are sold as such) have too much sugar or other sweetener such as malt. This usually conceals a basic lack of flavour, with slightly unpleasant chemical overtones.

Moisture

Moist loaves should retain their moist quality even when toasted. A good soda bread or pumpernickel will crisp on the outside but remain moist within, although it will dry out progressively. Bad bread steams visibly under the grill and becomes dry, like commercial crispbread.

Smell

The smell of bread should be seductive – nutty, wheaty, appealing. Bread that has no smell, or smells like toffee (common in industrial brown breads) is to be avoided.

WHAT'S BEST – BROWN OR WHITE?

Most British bread is made with **white** flour. This contains about 77–80 per cent of the wheat grain, with every last bit of the bran and wheatgerm removed. It can be either bleached (chemically whitened) or unbleached. White loaves with 'added fibre' have had softened grains added to white flour.

Brown bread is a pretty meaningless title. Most commercial 'brown' breads (such as Granary, Hi-Fibre, wheaten, malted oat, muesli and so on) are made with a high proportion of white flour to brown (see below), to which bran and wheatgerm particles have been added back in. Other ingredients are often included too, such as wheat or sunflower seeds. Caramel colour is sometimes used to give the bread a darker look. Some brown bread is also made with 'brown' flour. This has had the coarsest layers of the grain milled away and represents 85–95 per cent of the whole grain.

By law, **wholemeal** bread must be made with 100 per cent wholemeal flour. This includes the whole of the wheat grain with nothing taken away. A true wholemeal loaf should be labelled '100 per cent wholemeal'. Since nearly all the vitamins, minerals and fibre in wheat grain are concentrated in the outer layers, wholemeal flour is clearly much more nutritious than brown or white. By law, all white and brown loaves must be fortified with **vitamins** and **minerals** to replace some of those that have been removed by milling, but this does not mean that brown or white bread is as nutritious as 100 per cent wholemeal.

The nutritional advantage of eating bread made from wholemeal flour has to be balanced against the risks to human health posed by **pesticide residues**. Modern wheat is produced with a substantial chemical input in the form of fertilisers, pesticides and post-harvest chemical treatment in storage. Intensively produced cereals collect any residues from these treatments around the outside of the wheat grain – the bran. Considerably higher levels of residues are found in wholemeal flour and products made from it than in either brown or white flour. Certain highly toxic chemical inputs used in wheat production are known to survive both milling and baking.

As usual, there is no shortage of industry scientists and government experts to assure us that these residues are well within 'acceptable limits'. But these don't take into account the typical 'healthy eater', who consumes far more whole grains than the average British person. The clear alternative for those whose staple bread is wholemeal is to eat organic (see page 275).

TYPES OF WHEAT AND OTHER GRAINS FOR BREAD

Wheat is the most commonly used flour in breadmaking. It is graded according to its protein content. Wheats with a high protein content, known as **hard wheats**, are considered to be best for bread because the protein develops the strong gluten, which helps the dough rise easily. **Soft wheats** with less protein produce flour that is trickier to bake but often has a superior flavour to hard wheat. British and other European wheats tend to be relatively soft, while North American wheats are hard. The number of **wheat varieties** grown in Europe has reduced dramatically over the last few decades. While once varieties were selected for flavour, baking qualities, appropriateness to local growing circumstances and resistance to pests, modern varieties have been increasingly selected for early ripening and yield. Baking quality has become a secondary consideration, and taste has never figured.

A reaction against this loss of diversity has come with the rediscovery of more traditional varieties such as **Maris Widgeon, Flanders** and **Camp Remy**. These have a deeper, sweet-nutty flavour which underlines the one-dimensional qualities of standard modern varieties. More varieties like these are being taken up by progressive farmers, discerning millers and craft bakers. One such flour is **spelt**, a more nutritious precursor of wheat that until recently had almost disappeared. Other grains, such as **rye, oats, buckwheat** and **barley**, can all be incorporated into flour for bread but require more careful baking and produce heavier loaves because they do not have enough protein. So they are mainly used in combination with wheatflour. Flakes of grains, and seeds such as **sunflower, poppy and linseed**, can all be incorporated to give the bread special character and make it more nutritious.

Traditional **stoneground wheats and grains** are widely rated over modern roller-milled ones. Stoneground flours are slightly grittier and less porous than roller-milled ones because the stones grind the grain less finely. The grains do not become heated as they do with steel rollers. For these reasons, stoneground flours and grains (such as oats for porridge) generally have a more rounded flavour with plenty of texture and 'mouth-feel', as well as retaining more of their intrinsic nutrient goodness.

LEAVEN AND SOURDOUGH BREAD

Bread can be made without yeast. The raising ingredient is known as a leaven, or sourdough starter, and it is prepared by mixing flour and water, then allowing it to be colonised with wild yeasts that are naturally present in the flour and the atmosphere. It can also be made by keeping back a piece of dough from a previous batch of yeast bread, mixing that with flour and water, then leaving it to ferment.

Sourdough is the traditional style of bread eaten in Russia, Eastern Europe and Germany, usually in rye breads, and it is also very popular on the US West Coast. French country bread, *pain de campagne*, is traditionally made with *levain* (leaven). Even lighter, whiter breads such as baguette can be made with a proportion of leaven as well as some yeast.

Leaven gives the bread a distinctive sour, slightly tangy taste, which can be subtle or intense, depending on the baker's style. American sourdough bread is usually strong smelling and slightly vinegary, which does not appeal to everyone. French sourdoughs are generally more restrained, used in combination with whiter flours. All sourdough bread keeps quite well, and the flavour of the leaven becomes more pronounced as the bread ages.

Sourdough is more digestible than other bread because the bacteria in the leaven have already done some work on the flour starches before they reach the mouth. In the UK, sourdough bread has become more fashionable. Eastern European and Jewish bakeries have kept the tradition going and newer bakeries, committed to making bread by time-honoured techniques, have adopted this method. Industrial bakeries in the UK cannot cope with sourdough methods, although similar bakeries in other countries can. So if a baker produces sourdough bread, this is usually a good sign. It must be made patiently: non-'improved' flours, long periods of fermentation, traditional firing techniques and so on. It takes a little longer but the wait is usually worth it. Watch out for sourdough amateurs, though. Badly made sourdough bread is inedible!

Teas, Herbal and Fruit Infusions

If you are a typical tea drinker, the chances are you buy roughly the same sort of tea week in, week out. These days the vast bulk of tea we consume is in tea bags rather than loose. All we really know about it is that it looks black and produces a fairly standard amber brew.

This lack of knowledge is a rather sad state of affairs, since it means that we rarely get to appreciate the range of flavours and nuances that we lump under the general title of tea. What's even worse is that we may end up buying the most prosaic, basic-quality teas available, when there are many more interesting, and not necessarily more expensive, alternatives to try, if we only knew more about the subject.

The standard type of tea we commonly consume, either in bags, or loose, is **black tea**. Usually it comes from East Africa – Kenya and Malawi – and now to a lesser extent from the Indian sub-continent. Tea is produced in China (Keemun) and other countries throughout the world, too, but we import less from these sources.

Black tea is simply fresh green leaves and buds from the tea bush (*Camellia sinensis*), which have been withered, rolled, then allowed to ferment. Fermentation turns the tea black and it is then dried and sorted out into various grades. The tea is processed differently, depending on whether it is destined for tea bags or loose tea.

Assessing the quality of tea-bag tea

The tea inside the average tea bag is called C T C tea, which stands for 'cut, torn and curled'. The withered leaves are broken down mechanically into small pieces. This opens up the cell structure and means that the tea will brew more rapidly than whole-leaf tea. Most tea bags are blends of anything from 15 to 40 different teas, the blender's objective being to produce a standard, reliable product that will always be consistent. Teas alter from one harvest to the next, so the blend is changed to accommodate this, but always ensuring the favoured 'house style'.

All this coming and going makes it very difficult for consumers to assess the quality of tea in the bag. Very little hard information is given on the label. The finest teas are always sold loose rather than in tea bags but this does not mean that tea bags contain the worst available tea. As with loose tea, some is of a good standard in its category, some is terrible. You have to drink it, and inspect it closely, to find out.

There are two tests to apply. The first is colour. A good tea bag should produce brightly coloured tea with a nice red-orange hue. It should never look dull brown or have a grey tinge. The second is to break open the bag and look at the leaves once the tea has infused. They should have the same bright colour. If the tea is very compacted or dry, or has spots in it where the leaves have compacted into a wodge, it has not infused properly. This suggests that it contains too many poor-quality teas and tea dust.

Assessing the quality of loose black tea

Loose tea is known in the trade as **orthodox or classic tea**. Unlike C T C tea (see above), it is processed in a more traditional way and designed for slower infusion. The finest teas are sold in this way. There are three types.

Top grade is **whole-leaf tea**, where the leaves or buds are left intact. This is usually appreciated by those who like delicate teas. The tea is graded according to size of leaf, the most commonly encountered whole-leaf grade being **orange pekoe** – a technical term that has nothing to do with oranges. One step down comes **broken tea**, which, as its name suggests, has been either intentionally or unintentionally broken in harvesting or post-harvest handling. The most basic grade is what is known as **fannings**, tea that is so broken that it is in tiny bits, rather like coffee grounds. Both broken and fannings produce more full-bodied tea. With the exception of some fannings, which is sometimes so powdery that it is referred to, quite literally, as **tea dust**, all these grades are capable of producing fine tea, the difference being one of style rather than quality.

Although loose tea tends to be generally finer than tea bags, you need to be vigilant about what you are being sold. Packets of tea are frequently labelled with all sorts of meaningless names, such as 'fine', 'classic', 'connoisseur', 'choice', 'selected', 'speciality' and so on. Don't make the mistake of accepting these as a guarantee of quality. Equally, don't assume that when you choose an established brand name you are automatically buying quality. Buy your tea either in a specialist tea shop, which can give you precise, objective information on the grade you are buying, or in packets that have much more detailed labels.

Some very upmarket teas, such as the top Darjeelings, sell on the basis of their **estate name**. These are associated with quality but, like fine wines, they have both good and bad years. This is when blends are useful, because a skilled tea blender can balance various local teas to give the ideal qualities associated with that area. Unfortunately blends (for both tea bags and loose tea) are not properly regulated. In the UK a blend only has to contain 51 per cent of a named tea, so an Assam blend, for example, could quite legally contain 49 per cent of teas from non-Assam sources. Blends sold with a 'Darjeeling' label usually sport a **Darjeeling symbol**. Even though this symbol is sponsored by the Indian Tea

Board, it only guarantees that 60 per cent of the tea comes from Darjeeling!

TEA TALK TRANSLATED

There is a proliferation of technical trade terms for various types of black tea, indicated by mysterious letters after their name. India, for example, has a particular system for differentiating the type of leaf picked within the orange pekoe category. (A similar system operates for broken orange pekoe teas.) These are:

- SFTGFOP: special finest tippy golden flowery orange pekoe – finest FOP available
- FTGFOP: finest tippy golden flower orange pekoe – excellent-quality tea
- TGFOP: tippy golden flowery orange pekoe – contains a lot of golden buds
- GFOP: golden flowery orange pekoe – contains a smaller number of buds

Other tea-producing countries use terms such as 'pekoe', 'fannings', 'special', or 'superior', and variations on this system. Unfortunately for the consumer, such terms are not applied consistently from one country to another, or even from one tea estate to another, making them relatively useless as any sort of guide to quality.

Sri Lankan teas are classified in the same way, but also according to the altitudes at which they are grown:

- High-grown teas, which are planted at altitudes between 1200 and 2500 metres, are the most sought after. These are rated for finesse, producing a relatively light brew which is attractively perfumed
- Middle-grown teas (600–1200 metres) are richer, more rounded and have a deeper colour

> • Low-grown teas, grown at 600 metres or below, produce a dark, strong brew, which is sometimes very tannic. Most everyday Sri Lankan tea is of this type.
>
> Flush is simply the name given to a harvest, or picking, of tea. It is usually associated with teas from Darjeeling and Assam. First-flush teas are picked in the spring when the leaves are still young and green. Rare and precious, they are prized for their finesse and delicacy. Second-flush teas are picked in the summer, when the growth on the tea bushes is more vigorous. This produces teas that are deeper in colour, with a more pronounced, often fruity character. Third-flush teas are picked in the autumn, when the leaves are older and much larger. These teas are much darker in colour, richer and more aromatic.

GREEN TEA

Green tea, often called **Sencha**, is very different from the black tea most people drink. The standard brew in countries like China and Japan, it is simply green leaves that have been dried without being encouraged to ferment. Unlike black tea, green tea is nearly always sold as whole leaves or a powder.

Gunpowder tea is small, rolled-up balls of younger leaves. **Imperial** is a larger, looser version of gunpowder, and **Hyson** types are longer curled leaves which can be of different ages. There are no quality grades as such, but it would be a mistake to assume that green tea is poor quality. One of the most precious teas in the world is a green tea called **Gyokuro**. This sort of tea is almost revered in Japan where it is grown, the tea garden shaded with black curtains for three weeks pre-harvest so that the tea contains the maximum chlorophyll and minimum tannin. Teas produced by these prestigious tea gardens are sold on their name, but for other green teas price, unfortunately, is the only indicator of quality.

In the West, green tea is very underrated and underused. This is probably because it is drunk without milk or sugar, unlike the staple British black tea. Most people only come across it in the form of **jasmine tea**, which is either green or oolong tea with fresh jasmine leaves added. That is a pity, because green tea has two very attractive plus points as well as being delicious. The first is that it contains very little caffeine compared to other teas, so it is more calming and will not interfere with sleep. The second is that it is an extremely healthy drink, since it is a rich source of vitamins C, B1, B2, and E, as well as health-giving trace elements such as potassium, manganese, copper and zinc. Amongst other things, green tea is meant to be beneficial in aiding the flow of blood, encouraging digestion, easing water retention and hypertension, and even preventing tooth decay.

Unless you are lucky enough to have a really excellent specialist tea shop nearby, you are most likely to find green teas in health-food and natural food stores or Oriental food markets. Most supermarkets and even run-of-the-mill tea shops do not stock them.

OOLONG TEA

Oolong teas come from China, Japan and Formosa and are half-way between green and black tea. The green tea is allowed to ferment but not until it becomes a full-blown black tea. There are two types of oolong tea: **Chinese style**, where the fermentation is very short, and **Formosa style**, where the tea is allowed to ferment longer and produce a brew that is much closer to black tea. Because it is sold with leaves intact, oolong tea has no special grades, just geographical distinctions.

Oolong tea can be very subtle, light and refreshing. Like green tea, it is drunk on its own and contains almost no caffeine.

SOME UNUSUAL TEAS

White tea is a very rare and extremely expensive type of Chinese tea which undergoes no fermentation and consists of special silver-white buds. The most famous white tea in the world is called **Yin Zhen**, translated as 'silver needles'. This is a real collector's item, sought after for its pale mandarin colour and subtle perfume of buds.

Red tea is just another name for a tisane drunk extensively in South Africa known as Rooibos tea. It is not strictly a tea, since it comes from a different plant (*Aspalanthus linearis*). This kind of tea is very affordable and produces a refreshing, herbaceous brew that is totally caffeine free and very low in tannin, making it extremely mellow.

PERFUMED TEA

Any kind of tea – black, green or oolong – can be perfumed to lend it a special character. Traditional perfumed teas include **jasmine** (green tea scented with jasmine blossom), **Earl Grey** (black tea scented with citrussy bergamot oil or, occasionally, neroli oil) and **Lapsang Souchong** type (black tea smoked over woods such as spruce). These days, the majority of perfumed teas, such as Earl Grey, are scented not with natural oils but with **nature-identical flavourings**. These can vary in their make-up. Some are combinations of natural essential oils which, when blended, have a similar character to the real thing. Others contain a high proportion of flavour components that have been made in a laboratory. The rule is that if more than 95 per cent of the flavouring comes from a natural source it can be labelled as natural.

Nature-identical flavours have a longer shelf life than natural ones and are therefore very attractive to manufacturers. If your tea label lists just 'bergamot flavouring', it is likely to be nature-identical; if it says 'natural bergamot oil', it's the real thing. Natural oils oxidise more quickly than artificial ones, though they will still last for several years if stored correctly away from heat and light.

Since the 1970s, it has become increasingly fashionable to flavour or perfume black teas with aromatic oils, extracts and scented flowers. So you can now buy anything from mango tea, through chocolate and mint to 'Christmas tea', which is perfumed with cloves, orange zest and evocative spices. Some of these teas can be quite pleasant. But while some perfumed blends are actually quite upmarket products, using relatively expensive natural essences, oils, zests and other aromatics, others are low-quality black teas, flavoured with very dominant and unpleasant artificial aromas. These will be marked 'flavouring' on the list of contents. Avoid them like the plague!

THE SCENT OF TEA

You can tell quite a lot about tea by sniffing it – standard practice in top tea shops. First of all, you can discover if it smells fresh. Tea that has no scent, or smells dull or dank, is probably too old. Loose tea stays fresh for years if correctly stored in a dark, dry, airtight tin. Glass jars, light, extreme heat and damp are bad for tea.

All good tea should have its own individual character – something that is often clearer if you sniff your way around several teas in the same category. Oolong and green teas tend to smell more perfumed than black teas even if they have not been scented or had anything added. But even with black teas, it should be possible to pick out a style and aroma that please you.

TIME FOR TEA

When you see **breakfast** on a tea label, this usually indicates a blend that is full bodied, relatively acidic and tannic, and likely to wake you up. It tends to be broken teas from East Africa.

Afternoon or five o'clock tea, on the other hand, is more likely to be a whole-leaf tea with a higher proportion of more refined high-altitude, or F.O.P teas (see page 199).

203

Evening teas are usually green or oolong and therefore low in tannin.

None of these terms is defined by law, just custom and practice in the tea trade, so 'time-of-day' blends vary wildly from one tea merchant or label to another.

Tea production and workers' conditions

The tea industry has a bad reputation for the exploitation of tea pickers. According to the charity Christian Aid, tea pickers in Sri Lanka (nearly always women, often impoverished migrant labourers) may receive as little as 70 pence a day for what is a long and arduous task. Illiterate children frequently work alongside their parents as pickers in tea 'gardens' which, despite the name, are often run along plantation lines. This means that workers often have poor-quality, temporary living conditions and no social guarantees such as contracts, sick pay and so on.

Conditions vary according to the country of production and the type of employer. Apart from Kenya, where 50 per cent of tea is produced by small, independent farmers, most other tea production is either government controlled or owned by large transnational companies.

Very little tea is sold direct from the tea garden or estate, or packed there. Nearly all of it is sold through an auction system, which allows traders and middlemen to make more money from the gap between the producer and the consumer. Wholesalers in the West can make profits from the packaging and labelling of teas, thus allowing them to 'add value' to the basic product. Because tea producers are so remote, it is very difficult for consumers in the West to have any clear idea of how the tea they buy is produced. It is bought by our retailers at the tail-end of a long and complicated route, often involving sub-contracting deals.

Some of the large transnational companies involved in tea production are reacting to consumer concern over workers' conditions and introducing more egalitarian employment policies for their subsidiary companies to follow. Concerned consumers can look out for, and actively support, teas with a 'people-friendly' guarantee – labels such as Oxfam, Equal Exchange, Fairtrade and Traidcraft. In this way you can be sure that the tea you buy has been produced without exploitation of the workers and is socially, economically and environmentally sustainable. By supporting teas that offer this guarantee, consumers can put pressure on the handful of large, transnational companies that are active in tea production to put their house in order.

CHANGES BREWING

A wind of change is blowing through the world's tea-growing regions, many of which are converting their production to organic methods. Chemicals used in tea cultivation have become very expensive and have gradually ruined the soil, causing widespread soil erosion and influx of chemicals into rivers. High costs, combined with the low price of tea in international commodity trading, have made it hard for farmers to grow the crop profitably. Increasingly, they are seeing organic production as the solution.

In Sri Lanka, for example, the State Plantations Corporation (SLSPC) says: 'Conventional farming systems which are based on external inputs such as pesticides and fertilisers cannot offer all the solutions to our agricultural problems as we once hoped.' So the SLSPC is establishing an organic system which sustains production within a stable ecosystem and is not dependent on costly external inputs. This involves using natural fertilisers and insecticides, planting trees to 'fix' the nitrogen in the soil and prevent soil erosion, different pruning methods, tighter controls against pollution, and energy saving in tea processing.

Organic teas are increasingly available in the UK, at prices that are not significantly higher than conventional teas. You will find them in good supermarkets, health-food stores and Oxfam shops.

Herbal, fruit and flower infusions

Infusions – or what the French refer to as tisanes – are often simply lumped in with the general category of tea. This is pretty misleading for, with the exception of black teas that have been perfumed with herbs or fruits (see page 202), infusions have nothing whatsoever to do with tea. While all teas come from the same plant (*Camellia sinensis*), herbal and fruit infusions can be made from a variety of different plants, such as nettles, mint and verbena, or from fruit and flowers such as rosehip, elderflower, chamomile and so on.

Infusions have two good points in their favour straight away. The first is that they contain no caffeine, and so are attractive to people who have difficulty relaxing or sleeping. The second is that, in theory anyway, they are quasi-medicinal – that is, as well as being good to drink they have positively beneficial effects on your body. Chamomile, for example, is thought to have calming and soothing properties, so it is recommended for sleeping difficulties. Peppermint is meant to soothe wind and aid digestion. Lavender is prized for its mild antiseptic and anti-inflammatory qualities and so recommended for colds and sinusitius.

There is no doubt that plants do have medicinal properties, but the law at present prevents manufacturers making any such claims for infusions. This is just as well, for to have the effects we associate with them the infusions must contain herbs or flowers that are of **pharmaceutical standard**. That just means that they contain enough of the essential oils that give the plant its characteristic properties to be used as medicines.

Unless an infusion is labelled 'pharmaceutical grade' – and these are few and far between – it is best to think of them as just pleasant-tasting drinks which make a good alternative to tea or coffee, and might possibly have some desirable effects. As with black tea, most infusions are sold in tea-bag form, and the quality (and freshness) of the contents is anyone's guess. There are more and more infusions on sale with fanciful names and pungent perfumes, many of which contain a natural herb or plant base that has been liberally dosed with cheap and nasty artificial flavourings.

As with perfumed black teas, go for brands that give you some detailed information about their quality. If you like flavoured infusions, choose ones that use natural essences and aromas rather than artificial ones. The latter are easy to spot because they smell like cheap fruit pastilles or scented soap.

Last but not least, it is worth remembering that you don't *need* to buy infusions in tea-bag form. Herbal, fruit and flower infusions are simple to make at home and usually much better. After all, they are only boiling water poured on the plant of your choice and allowed to brew. One point worth bearing in mind, though, is that fresh herbs taste much better than dried ones, whether these come loose from a shop or in tea-bag form. Like spices, herbs sold loose for infusion often suffer badly for want of a sell-by date, rapidly losing their freshness. If you buy fresh herbs, you can instantly see the quality of what you are getting. Try comparing an infusion made with fresh mint leaves against a mint tea bag if you are not convinced!

Coffee

Around 90 per cent of the coffee drunk in the UK is instant. This marks us out from other Europeans and from Americans, who favour roast and ground coffees. It is fair to say that we appear to be addicted to the stuff.

Amongst coffee lovers, instant has a poor reputation. Whether you rate it or not, there is no doubt that no instant coffee tastes anything like freshly made roast and ground coffee. Obviously a lot of people think that instant coffee has its uses. It is certainly convenient. But the frustrating thing is that instant – even allowing for recent improvements such as the increased use of arabica beans – is a most unsatisfactory way to taste the potential of coffee.

If the majority of consumers realise that, fair enough. However, the vast advertising budgets that are pumped into promoting instant coffee make it sound as though it was the best in the world. Adverts consistently blur the distinction between instant and ground coffee as though they were one and the same. And that's a con! Discovering 'real' ground coffee is one of life's great pleasures (see page 215). Drink instant out of laziness or pragmatism if you must, but don't be under any illusions about what you are getting.

Instant coffee

Instant coffee was developed as a wartime 'dry' supply for the American forces. Its base is liquid coffee – coffee that has already been brewed.

The original method of producing it is to evaporate the liquid coffee in tall, chimney-type towers by using a hot current of air. This produces a thick spray of dried coffee particles which fall to the bottom. The second, more favoured modern approach is freeze drying. This produces better coffee because it conserves more of the subtle aromas.

Both methods are entirely industrial, involving the brewing of huge vats of coffee in vast processing plants. Traditionally, the quality of the basic coffee used for instant was fairly low, as befits a second-best product designed for convenience.

Amongst the world's coffees, there is a two-way quality split. **Arabica coffees** are the best. These grow typically in high-altitude areas (above 610 metres). They are, however, more fragile and less prolific than the vigorous and high-yielding **robusta coffees**, which grow in lower areas (below 610 metres). Robusta coffees are grown in many countries around the world and are coarser and less aromatic than arabicas. The bulk of instant coffee is made from these cheaper, less-desirable beans.

IMPROVING INSTANT COFFEE

As instant coffee has assumed its position as the main type of coffee that most people drink, coffee manufacturers have tried to improve standards. In addition to making freeze-dried coffee, which has largely overtaken instant powder in popularity, more producers are making play of the fact that they use exclusively arabica coffees, or at least a high proportion of these. Although this change in emphasis has improved the quality of instant coffee and helped to give it a more upmarket image, it is an improvement from a very low base. While robustas are inferior coffees, undistinguished arabicas may be little better. As with all commercial blends, coffee manufacturers offer consumers no hard information on the origins or grade of the coffee.

It is common to see brands sold by the name of the country, such as Colombian. This is about as useful as being told that an apple is green as opposed to red. It is invariably accompanied by meaningless assurances about being 'carefully blended' to preserve the characteristics of this very special coffee and so on.

Be sceptical. Even arabica instant coffees can be made with bulk beans, produced with no particular regard for quality.

Ground coffee and coffee beans

If you buy fresh coffee you have a choice, depending on how far your interest in it extends. You can either go for standard brands or find a specialist source with a more interesting range.

COMMERCIAL BRANDS OF GROUND COFFEE AND BEANS

These are the big-name brands available in all supermarkets and shops. These days most are arabica beans, but a few blends may still have a proportion of robusta added. So only buy coffees labelled 'All Arabica', unless you actively favour the coarse, rubbery, scorched-tyres flavour of robusta coffee in espresso blends (see page 216).

The most striking thing about the standard ground coffees and beans on sale is the almost total absence of any specific information about their quality. These coffees are usually described in one of two ways. Like instant coffee, some are labelled according to country. Others are sold by the type of roast and are mainly blends – Continental (dark roast), breakfast (medium roast), espresso (high roast). Also like instant coffee, all this is usually accompanied by a load of waffle about 'master roasters', 'skilled blending' and 'careful selection from high-altitude plantations'.

While many of these coffees are of fair to very reasonable quality, this anonymous way of selling them does nothing to inform us or to heighten our appreciation of what we are getting. It's a bit like buying a piece of meat marked 'Scottish Sunday Joint – carefully prepared by a master butcher'. Few of us would find that lack of objective information very satisfactory!

If you buy these commercial brands often, make a point of comparing them with coffee bought freshly roasted from a well-chosen specialist coffee shop. The chances are you can get a better coffee there for the same price.

THE BEST PACKAGING AND STORAGE FOR COFFEE

Since coffee (especially ground), rapidly loses its freshness and becomes stale, it is best to buy brands that are sold, not in rigid packs or tins, but in more flexible packs with what is known as a freshness valve.

After coffee has been roasted it gives off carbon dioxide, so many manufacturers allow the ground coffee to 'de-gas' for a few days before packing. Unfortunately, this means the coffee also loses many of the aromatic elements that give it its flavour and aroma. The volatile oils that remain oxidise, and the coffee goes stale rapidly. Freshness valves are devices that enable the carbon dioxide gas to escape, allowing air back in. This means that the coffee can be packed right after it is roasted and ground, making it much fresher. Most high-quality commercial coffees are packed by this method now.

Once you get them home, coffee beans are best used quickly or stored in the freezer. Ground coffee should be put in a dark, airtight tin and used quickly – preferably within a week. Ground coffee and, to a lesser extent, beans, deteriorate when exposed to heat, air and light.

FINDING A GOOD COFFEE SHOP

If you want to go beyond the anonymity of commercial coffee blends, look for a specialist coffee shop which buys in its own beans and roasts them. Other shops, such as small delicatessens, buy in coffee from the nearest coffee wholesaler. Make sure they have a rapid turnover, because coffee deteriorates quickly once roasted, so a brisk trade is essential. Avoid shops displaying coffee in glass jars. A roasted bean is only good for six weeks, and heat and light cause oxidation.

Roasting coffee is one of the most seductive aromas imaginable, so it is tempting to assume that every bean from that shop will be equally delicious. Not so. There are very marked differences in types of beans and roasts. Pay attention to what you are buying so that your tasting experience will leave you more informed for future purchases. As with all good food shops, staff should be very knowledgeable about their subject, and happy to talk you through the various coffees.

COFFEE TALK TRANSLATED

Coffee labels are peppered with words and descriptions often incomprehensible to the consumer. Here's the lowdown on the vocabulary you will encounter.

After picking, coffee beans need to be removed from their outer layer or husk. There are two ways of doing this. When water is used these are called **washed coffees**. After soaking, the wet husk is removed with rollers. This type of treatment is thought to be superior to **dry coffees** or **naturals**, where the ripe coffee **cherries** (as unhulled beans are known) are merely left in the sun to loosen the husk. This is because washed coffees are slightly fermented before washing, which is thought to add to their flavour.

One particularly delicious treatment is a process known as **Monsooning**, which is used for Indian **Mysore** coffee. After it has been washed and hulled, the coffee is laid out on racks and dried naturally by coastal monsoon winds. The beans take on a soft, golden colour, producing a coffee which is rich, low in acidity, and has an intriguingly complex flavour. A real collector's coffee.

Aged coffees, such as **Old Matured Java**, take on a deeper, more rounded flavour, while retaining considerable strength and body. **New crop** coffees can be more 'grassy' and with more herbaceous acid than aged ones. Ageing decreases acidity.

Coffee 'cherries' usually contain two beans. Some have just one and are referred to as **peaberries**. Peaberry coffee is thought to have a more concentrated flavour.

AA or Double A beans are very uniform beans which roast very evenly. However, this is a grading on appearance only, not overall quality. It usually describes Kenyan and other East African coffees. **Longberry** and **shortberry**, too, are simply trade terms for describing the beans' shape and not an indicator of quality. **Maragogype** is an outsized mutant Mexican bean, popular more for its appearance than its flavour.

Although 'mocha' is widely used in cooking to refer to a combination of coffee and chocolate, **Mocha** beans have nothing to do with chocolate. It is a term used to describe coffees from Ethiopia and the Yemen, the name taken from the Yemeni city of Al Makha, which is meant to be the source of the world's first coffee.

DISTINGUISHING SINGLE-ORIGIN COFFEES AND BLENDS

It is really important to keep in your mind the distinction between single-origin coffees (originals) and blends. As a rule of thumb, you can judge the excellence of a coffee shop by the number of original arabica coffees it has. These are beans from one specific source, which have not been blended already. A good coffee shop should be selling far more single-origin coffees than blends.

Blends from good specialist shops can be excellent, though, and blending is an art. While single-origin coffees might vary in quality from year to year, a house blend should offer you continuity, balance and reliability.

Single-origin coffees, however, remain the first division of the world's coffee production. They are of such distinguished quality that they are generally sold unblended for drinking on their own. More workaday arabicas (and the cheaper robustas in commercial brands) usually find their way into blends. By combining coffees with different characteristics and qualities, blenders can make reasonable, if never outstanding, drinks.

Obviously, in the hands of a skilled blender of high-quality coffees, some blends can be marvellous. High-quality single-origin coffees can be blended to produce a coffee that is perfectly adapted to certain tastes and requirements. However, although coffee blend-ing is a totally honourable activity in principle, it does allow for more liberties to be taken when it comes to the quality of the basic coffee.

Because 'house blends' are often cheaper than single-origin coffees they can seem very tempting. They can work out cheaper simply because the shop sells a lot of them. But if you buy blends, select ones that offer the maximum of hard information about their contents. A blend labelled 'Viennese After Dinner' or 'Best Brazilian' without any other supplementary information could be anything. You haven't got a clue what you are getting, and you certainly are not going to learn much about the differences between coffees by drinking it.

Some blends are actively misleading. Take those familiar 'mountain blends'. These often exploit the cachet surrounding the single-source and relatively rare Jamaican Blue Mountain coffee (see page 220) in order to sell a much more ordinary blend of undistinguished beans. A good blend should state the individual origins of each coffee within it. For example 'After Dinner – a blend of mellow Indonesian Java with spicy Indian Mysore, roasted dark'. Blends made from excellent single-origin coffees have no reason to hide their source from the consumer.

CHECKING THE STATE OF THE BEANS

Whether you choose a blend or a single-origin coffee, have a good look at the beans before you buy or grind them. Robusta beans look small and mean compared to arabica, so it is easy to spot them. Robusta coffee has no place in a really good coffee shop except in high-roast espresso blends.

Arabica beans vary in shape and size from one source to another but it is important that they look smooth and intact, not broken, bitty or scruffy. This is a sign of poor handling and quality control. Look for nice, smooth, even beans with the minimum of imperfections.

FINDING YOUR WAY AROUND SINGLE-ORIGIN COFFEES

Selecting fine coffee is a fascinating, but often baffling experience. It is easy to see why, when presented with a selection of, say, 20 single-origin coffees, many consumers tend to identify one they like, or like the sound of, and stick to it. However, there are certain characteristics by which many disparate coffees can be grouped. Once you know this you can build up a clearer picture of what you like in a coffee, and the areas of the world that are most likely to provide it.

Coffee comes from a variety of countries around the world

which lie, more or less, between the tropic of Cancer and the tropic of Capricorn. The country alone is no guarantee of quality. Brazil, for example, produces 30 per cent of the world's coffee. But with the exception of Santos (see the chart on page 218), most of these are not particularly distinguished.

The best arabicas – like fine teas – come from high-altitude locations. These conditions favour the fickle varieties of arabica coffee tree which produce the most aromatic and complex beans.

Single-source coffees are all subtly different, and very difficult to describe. To make the subject even more complicated, just like grapes for wine, the flavour and quality can vary from year to year, depending on weather, political upheavals, market price and so on.

The most useful initial way of sorting them out is by their 'body' – some coffees are naturally more heavy in the mouth, seeming full bodied in relation to others which are 'thin'. Thereafter, certain other classifications can be applied. Some coffees tend to be more neutral while others are 'aromatic'. This means it has a particular character, fragrance or flavour, which varies with each type of coffee. All coffees contain acid but some are noticeably more acidic (like the acid when it is allied with fruitiness in white wine) than others. All this is not a question of good versus bad, simply preference.

The coffee world can be roughly divided into three areas:

- **The Caribbean and Central and South America**
  The better coffees from this area are generally smooth and well-balanced, with no single element predominating. Flavour, acidity and body all live together harmoniously, which is why they are sometimes called by the rather misleading term, mild. In countries such as Mexico and Nicaragua, the acidity can tend to be metallic in some cases, and the body thin.

- **East Africa and Arabia**
  These coffees have a pronounced acidity, most evident in the better-quality Kenyans. At best, this acidity is a distinctive fruitiness, akin to that of a dry white wine. At worst, such as in low-

quality Malawi coffees, the acidity turns into a grassy harshness. In the classic Yemeni coffee and some unwashed Ethiopians, a pleasant 'off' or 'high' note reminiscent of game or cheese is discernible.

- **India, Southeast Asia and the Pacific**
Smoothness, low acidity and heavy body broadly characterise coffees from this region. High-quality Java and Sumatra coffees have a very heavy body, sometimes accentuated by ageing. In poorer qualities, an unpleasant earthy note creeps in.

There are numerous mavericks which fail to meet these generalisations, and some of these appear in the table on the following page.

FINDING THE ROASTING STYLE YOU LIKE

Unroasted or 'green' coffee beans start out pale khaki, like the colour of putty, and are flavourless. The skill of the roaster lies in roasting them just enough to extract all the flavours of each coffee type, bringing out their characteristic tastes and aromas. The degree of roasting should usually relate to the basic strength of the coffee. While a full-bodied coffee may stand up to a fairly dark roast, this would be too heavy-handed for a delicate coffee such as Brazilian Santos, which would be better mild to medium roasted. Over-roasting destroys the balance of flavour in the beans. Most single-origin coffees are therefore only medium roasted. In good house blends, each different type of bean in the blend should have been individually roasted before mixing. Roasting also has the effect of driving off all or most of the acids in a coffee, carbonising the beans and producing a more bitter flavour.

Care should be taken when buying dark roasts. Though this is a very popular style for coffee in many countries, it is also easier to disguise poorer quality arabica and robusta coffees by very dark roasting. Many dark-roasted coffees are actually burnt, giving the coffee an additional strength and body not matched by flavour. The flavour may have been roasted out.

A GUIDE TO SINGLE-ORIGIN COFFEES

All coffees are given a score from 1–5 in each of the three areas of flavour, body and acidity. A score of 1 in the body column will mean a thin coffee, 5 a rich body, and so on.

Country	Type	Flavour	Body	Acidity
Caribbean, Central and South America				
Brazil	Santos	2	2	2
Columbia	Supremo	4	3	3
	Medellin Excelso	2	3	2
Peru	Chanchamayo	2	2	2
Mexico	Maragogype	2	1	3
El Salvador	(no varietal name)	3	3	3
Honduras	(no varietal name)	2	3	2
Guatamala	Antigua	3	3	3
Costa Rica	Tarrazu, Tres Rios	3	3	3
Jamaica	Blue Mountain	5	3	3
Cuba	Escambray	3	3	2
Puerto Rico	Yauco Selecto	3	3	3

East Africa and Arabia

Region	Variety		
Kenya	AA Peaberry	5	4
Ethiopia	Djimma (unwashed)	2	2
	Harrar Longberry, Sidamo, Yergacheffe (all washed)	4	4
Yemen	Mattari, Ismaili	5	3
Tanzania	Kibu Chagga	3	4
Zimbabwe	(no varietal name)	4	3

India, Southeast Asia and the Pacific

Region	Variety		
India	Mysore	3	2
	Monsooned Malabar	4	2
Sumatra	DP	2	1
	Mandheling	4	2
Java	Old Brown	4	1
New Guinea	Plantation X	4	4
Celebes	Kalossi	4	3
Hawaii	Kona	3	3

Others

Region	Variety		
Saint Helena	(no varietal name)	5	3

Common roasting styles and terminology

Light- and medium-roast coffees are not always labelled as such but you can pick them out by the comparative colour of the bean – they look browner and less black than others. This is sometimes also referred to unhelpfully as a Dutch roast.

Dark- or full-roast coffees are generally labelled as Continental, French or Viennese (when fig is added).

Heavily roast coffees are sold as espresso.

FINDING THE RIGHT GRIND

Pulverised coffee is what you need to make Turkish or Greek coffee, using preferably Yemeni but frequently Brazilian beans, lightly roasted.

Very fine-ground coffee is best for electric espresso machines and paper filter methods.

Fine-ground coffee is best for cafetières (plunger), two-tiered Italian coffee pots (stovetop espressos), glass cona and 'drip pots'.

Medium-ground coffee is recommended for the traditional 'jug' method and percolators.

PRICE AS A GUIDE TO QUALITY

In the main, the price of coffee is a reasonable guide to quality. Cheaper coffees tend to be rather ordinary blends and, in terms of value for money, they often represent poor quality. Most widely available single-origin arabica coffees are affordable and may even work out cheaper than instant coffee, which is actually a very pricy product, even though it is made from cheaper beans.

Certain rare coffees are collector's items. Some are moderately expensive when available while others, mainly very small crops, have obtained a sort of sacred status and become accordingly exceptionally expensive. The best examples of this are Hawaiian Kona and Jamaican Blue Mountain. Though these are very fine coffees, it is doubtful that their inflated price tag can be justified when you separate the quality from the hype.

There are many much cheaper coffees available which can match these in quality. If you want the best value for money, bypass the cheap and the very expensive and look to middle-priced coffees.

FLAVOURED COFFEES

Amaretto, After Eight, Whisky, Chocolate Truffle – just some of the new 'flavoured' coffees that have come on the market over the last decade. Unlike tea and chocolate, which have a noble history of partnering with a range of natural flavours and scents, coffee has no such pedigree. Most coffees are flavoured with actively unpleasant artificial aromas and even on the rare occasions where natural flavourings are used they do not combine well with coffee. Flavoured coffee is a modern gimmick. Even if the basic coffee was any good, you wouldn't be able to taste it. If you want to know what coffee tastes like when partnered with chocolate, praline or any of the other coffee 'flavours' around, try making a pudding!

Certain very traditional coffees drunk in countries such as France have chicory or roasted barley added. This is a cheaper way of giving coffee a bitter flavour and not recommended.

Some Viennese blends have fig added to lend a touch of sweetness and richness – an acquired taste.

THE BEST DECAFFEINATED COFFEE

Most decaffeinated coffee is made by the least desirable process, the **solvent method**. This involves steaming the unroasted beans, then soaking them in a chemical solvent to remove the caffeine. The safety of chemical solvents in food is questionable. Certain solvents that were previously used for coffee decaffeinating have been banned because they were either carcinogenic or environmentally unfriendly. Various refinements on more benevolent chemical solvent methods are being tried out but there is still a risk of residues being left behind in the coffee. Unless a decaffeinated coffee is labelled explicitly to the contrary, it is reasonable to assume that it is made by a solvent method.

A much healthier and more natural method is known as the **water method**. There are different variations. One is soaking the beans in water containing a low concentration of caffeine. This acts as a magnet, encouraging the extraction of caffeine from the beans. Another is filtering the caffeine from the water using charcoal.

A third approach is the **carbon dioxide method**, where beans are soaked in liquid and gas carbon dioxide which combines with the caffeine. Though this is more technological than water, it appears to pose no risk to human health and produces coffee with a more concentrated flavour than water-process coffee.

Both water-process and CO_2-process coffees are generally more expensive than those decaffeinated with solvents.

It is very difficult to find water, or CO_2-method decaffeinated coffee in large stores but they should be standard in specialist coffee shops and healthfood stores. Irrespective of the decaffeination method, most decaffeinated coffees taste somehow feeble, as though something was lacking. Coffee lovers with sleeping problems may ultimately find more to satisfy them in herbal infusions (see page 206).

Cup for cup, instant coffee contains less caffeine than freshly made ground coffee. Arabica coffees contain less caffeine than robustas. The higher-grown the arabica, the less caffeine. Similar-altitude arabica coffees also contain different levels of caffeine – Brazilian Santos, for example, is relatively low in caffeine, while Ethiopian Harrar is naturally stronger. A good specialist coffee merchant should be able to advise you about this.

ORGANIC COFFEES

More organic coffees – coffees produced without the aid of chemical fertilisers and pesticides – are coming on to the market. Over-use of chemicals is an acknowledged problem in coffee production, a problem exacerbated by the fact that coffee-producing countries still use many highly toxic chemicals that have been banned, or have had their uses seriously limited, in Europe.

Because much coffee is grown as a cash crop by poor rural workers living on the breadline, quality control is not always very strict. Many peasant farmers are illiterate and cannot read the instructions for applying chemical treatments to coffee trees. As a result, stipulations as to what protective clothing should be worn, periods to be observed before harvesting after chemical treatment and so on, are often ignored. For growers whose financial security is perilous, the temptation to over-use chemicals to disguise disease problems in a crop can be irresistible.

For European buyers, controls on the use of chemicals are difficult to enforce and check, since coffee from one country is often pulled together from several sources by regional collectors, sold through state marketing boards, then bought on a world market, through many intermediaries.

Organic coffee production has not died out in certain traditional coffee-producing countries and some of the finest arabica coffees are carefully produced by low-input, even strictly organic methods. Organic is becoming more popular amongst more progressive, forward-thinking producers.

MAX HAVELAAR AND FAIR-TRADE COFFEES

The idea of fair-trade coffees took off in 1989 in Holland. A new 'Max Havelaar' seal of approval was introduced to delineate coffees that had been traded in such a way as to give producers a much better deal. The name came from an influential 19th-century Dutch novel in which the central character, Max Havelaar, recounts the terrible conditions in what was then the Dutch colony of Indonesia.

Though colonial-style slave labour is a thing of the past, many coffee producers still live in a cycle of deprivation and poverty, which is due, at least in part, to the way the rest of the world trades with them. Typical coffee workers are small peasant farmers, who lack the financial security to set up the sort of local infrastructure necessary to market what they produce. This means that they mainly sell what they grow to middlemen and agents and so miss out on the lucrative 'value-added' activities surrounding coffee – grinding, roasting, processing and packaging – which are carried out elsewhere. To make matters worse, coffee prices are notoriously volatile, which leaves small farmers at the whim of world markets, often having to sell their production for less than it is worth.

Inspired by the Max Havelaar initiative, a number of different fair-trade schemes have been set up in the UK. Under these schemes, which sell under labels such as **Cafédirect, Oxfam, Traidcraft** and **Fairtrade Foundation**, European buyers enter into direct trading with producers. Coffee prices, which are anything from 10–100 per cent above the market rate, are set in advance and are honoured irrespective of world prices. Cash is often paid in advance and producers are given advantageous credit arrangements and long-term contractual commitment.

Many fair-trade coffees are organic. Those which are not are grown in an environmentally friendly way. In practical terms, this means that certain pesticides widely used in coffee production are banned and that alternative (non-chemical) means of pest control are being developed. In addition, standards must include safeguards against water pollution and protection of forested areas. This all ensures that coffee cultivation is carried out on a sustainable basis, leaving no environmental damage for future generations.

Fair-trade schemes give coffee growers the precious capital and financial stability they need. They can mean schools for those who have never had the chance of education, healthcare centres, better water facilities, a new packaging plant – whatever improves life.

For consumers, fair-trade coffee comes with a guarantee that workers have been paid to acceptable levels, that they enjoy basic healthcare and safety standards, and that the coffee has been produced in an environmentally friendly way.

Storecupboard and Fridge A–Z

This section lists the most common items and groups of food that you are likely to have in your kitchen which are not covered in other main sections.

Biscuits and cakes

The simplest way to select the best-quality biscuits and cakes is by paying attention to the ingredients listing. This should read like the ingredients required for a comparable recipe you would make at home: flour, butter, sugar, eggs, natural vanilla and so on. If the ingredients listing runs on at length and includes items you haven't heard of or whose function you don't recognise, such as whey, hydrogenated fat, glucose, milk powder, flavourings, emulsifiers, stabilisers and colours, then you have probably got a packet of over-processed junk on your hands.

Beyond that, favour products that show some signs of awareness of the quality of ingredients, such as 'stoneground flour', 'unrefined cane sugar', 'natural extract of vanilla', 'eggs freshly cracked at time of preparation', 'organic wheatflour', 'sea salt', 'unhydrogenated vegetable oil' and so on.

Breakfast cereals

The common British breakfast cereals, like the standard British sliced and wrapped loaf, are a good example of how the food industry loves to take a basically healthy food to pieces and put it back together again in a more profitable, but nutritionally compromised form.

The most modern **breakfast cereals marketed at children** generally contain similar levels of sugar to sweets and confectionery. The more **established breakfast cereals**, such as rice crispies and cornflakes, contain a lot less but are still surprisingly sweet, as you will notice if you go back and taste milk that has recently had some in it. The occasional sugar-free product in this category is generally so tasteless and devoid of character that it is hard to get it down – any sound flavours from wholesome cereals have long since been lost in the processing. Prominent additions of healthy vitamins (artificially produced) are peppered over the packaging to make you think that the product is good for you. But it is only fortified with vitamins because most of the goodness associated with the grain in its whole form has been milled and processed out!

Newer **muesli** products have recently come on the market. The **granola-types** are visibly stuck together with sugar (as are their offspring, cereal bars), generally in disguised, healthier-sounding forms such as honey, fructose and so on. Preferable though these sugars are to straight sucrose, many products that contain them are ridiculously sweet. 'No-added-sugar' versions generally achieve the overwhelming level of sweetness deemed necessary by adding lots of sweet fruits, such as raisins, dried banana and mango chips. Items like chocolate chips and fruit flavourings are creeping in and giving the game away. Better-quality muesli bases and individual grains can usually be bought in wholefood shops and are easy to mix and toast at home. Porridge oats, which are highly nutritious, are widely available. As with all whole grains, these are best stoneground and, preferably, organic (see Bread).

Chocolate, cocoa and drinking chocolate

Americans draw a distinction between candy and chocolate. Candy refers to items that may include chocolate in their preparation but usually contain lots of other ingredients – mainly sugar, fondant centres, caramel, vegetable fats, flavourings and so on. It is a pity that the UK does not make the same distinction because there is no doubt that many of us are heartily confused about what chocolate is.

The ingredients of the real thing – **dark chocolate** – are short and sweet: cocoa solids and cocoa butter, a small amount of sugar, and a tiny bit of lecithin (an emulsifier widely regarded as safe) to bind it. Often a drop of natural extract of vanilla is added as a flavouring.

As a general rule, the higher the proportion of cocoa solids, the better the chocolate. Less than a decade ago dark chocolate was considered high quality if it contained more than 30 per cent cocoa solids. Nowadays, as awareness of chocolate quality grows, a good dark chocolate is considered to be around 60 per cent and the best ones 70 per cent. Beyond that, the bitterness becomes too dominant for most tastes.

There are three types of beans used to make cocoa. The Forastero – the workaday cocoa bean – accounts for the bulk of world cocoa production. It is good and strong but not very aromatic. Trinitario and Criollo beans are less prolific and therefore cost more, but they have more intrinsic character. High-quality dark chocolate is made with all three, but Trinitario and Criollo remain the chocolate lover's first choice.

There are several ways to assess the quality of dark chocolate:
- **Appearance:** It should look smooth, shiny and mahogany-black.
- **Smell:** This should make your mouth water.
- **Sound:** The bar should make a distinct 'cracking' noise when you break it.
- **Texture:** This should be ultra smooth, melt-in-the-mouth, without graininess.

- **Taste:** This should be dark, rich, complex, long-lasting and fruity, with distinctive flavours (red fruit, tobacco, raisins) depending on the type of bean and where it has been grown.

Thereafter, the price of dark chocolate varies according to the care with which it has been made, the type of beans used and their origins.

Signs of poor-quality dark chocolate include gritty texture (chocolate made in a rush which has not been patiently 'conched', i.e. ground and smoothed); no 'crack' (a sign that vegetable fat has been included, see below); dull colour and white bloom (old or badly stored); and an unpleasantly bitter burnt flavour (the beans have been over-roasted, usually an attempt to lend character to mediocre beans). The use of artificial vanillin flavouring (see page 265) is always a bad sign. Even if this was good chocolate, the artificial flavour would ruin it.

There is good **milk chocolate** around, but it is not always easy to find. Most British milk chocolate contains about 20 per cent cocoa solids, which are all from Forastero beans. Up to 5 per cent vegetable fat is added to make the product cheaper. Vegetable fat does not have the natural melt-in-the-mouth qualities of cocoa butter, and leaves a greasy film on the roof of the mouth. Large quantities of undeclared white sugar are included in milk chocolate – up to 50 per cent is allowed by law. Artificial flavourings are commonly added.

Better-quality milk chocolate (usually from abroad) does not contain vegetable fat or artificial flavourings and has a much higher cocoa solids content of around 40 per cent.

White chocolate contains no cocoa solids, just cocoa butter. Otherwise, it usually contains the same additives as basic milk chocolate. Some specialist food shops sell good-quality white chocolate, the best of which is usually French.

Diet, or **low-calorie chocolate** is generally made by using vegetable fat up to the maximum and substituting artificial sweetener for sugar (see Sugar Substitutes). Both these ingredients are controversial on health grounds.

Chocolate that has been traded in such a way as to give producers a better deal is becoming more widely available. Look out for the **Fairtrade mark**. **Organic chocolate** is also making its presence felt in both wholefood shops and supermarkets. Cocoa production is widely recognised to be chemical intensive and inadequately regulated. Many cocoa workers labour without effective protection or safeguards in conditions that would not be tolerated in European countries.

Cocoa powder should have only one ingredient – cocoa – and no added sugar. The best cocoas are Dutch and French, since these are processed in such a way that the flavour is more intense and the covering qualities (for coating truffles and so on) are much better. Some cocoa powder sold in healthfood shops has had some of its fat removed, resulting in fewer calories but also less flavour.

Drinking chocolate and chocolate drinks sell on the fact that they are instant – just add milk and no blending. However, making cocoa the traditional way is a small effort for something that tastes infinitely better. Instant drinking chocolate and chocolate drinks routinely contain lots of sugar in several forms, powdered milk and whey, plus thickeners, emulsifiers and artificial flavourings in ever more outlandish guises. As usual, many justify a 'low-calorie' claim by the use of artificial sweetener instead of sugar. It is a conveniently limited way to look at the health and nutritional qualities of these highly processed and artificial products.

Crisps, potato and corn snacks

In their most basic form, there is nothing too terrible about **crisps**. They are just thin slices of potatoes fried in liquid vegetable fat, then dusted with salt. This makes them fatty and they carry quite a lot of salt because you eat them thin and you eat quite a few of them, but they do nevertheless retain quite a lot of the vitamin C that you would get in cooked potatoes.

The horrors creep in with 'flavour' crisps. Some flavours come from relatively natural, albeit heavily processed sources, such as dried tomato, cheese and onion powders, but the majority also contain unspecified artificial flavourings. There are literally thousands of these in use, but their toxicological effects are inadequately monitored.

A sweet flavour is deemed essential to flavoured crisps. This comes in the form of sugars such as lactose and dextrose and artificial sweeteners such as saccharin (see Sugar Substitutes). Another common type of additive is a flavour enhancer. Commonly used enhancers include yeast extract, monosodium glutamate and hydrolised vegetable protein (HVP). These are essentially amino acids which enhance other artificial flavours and give a sort of 'meaty' taste. HVP has now been taken out of commercial baby foods because of worries that it may affect growth and cause brain damage.

The **potato snacks** that come in shapes, not slices, are known as extruded snacks, since the mixture is forced out of a machine before frying. They have none of the limited virtues of crisps and tend to be made from a basic mix of dehydrated potato and potato starch, salt, emulsifiers and monosodium glutamate. The latter is widely used in cheap, processed foods and causes allergic reactions in some people. Flavoured versions of potato snacks contain the same motley ingredients as those used in crisps.

Corn tortilla chips are manufactured in a similar way to crisps. Even some apparently upmarket versions contain pretty downmarket additives and flavourings. Some wholefood shops sell organic tortilla chips made from blue corn, which is thought to be more nutritious than yellow corn.

Seemingly improved versions of crisps and snacks cannot always be trusted. Some of those claiming more traditional production methods are extremely high in fat. One brand's 'lower-fat' crisp can contain more fat than another brand's regular crisp. 'Light' or slimming versions often just use artificial sweeteners instead of sugar because they have fewer calories. These sorts of snacks need to be approached with a little common sense. The basic ones are fatty and salty, so it is not a good idea to eat them often. The flavoured ones won't just make you thirsty, they'll wreak havoc with your tastebuds and possibly your long-term health.

Dried and candied fruit

When selecting good-quality **dried fruit**, be they dates, sultanas, prunes, raisins, cherries or apricots, don't go for anonymous bags of mixed or vine fruits. These are usually miserable, gritty specimens. Choose individual fruits and buy the best you can afford, then mix them according to your needs. Favour those with a pedigree, from a specific region or of a certain named variety, such as Agen prunes or Lexia raisins. These are likely to be better than the standard, unspecific equivalent.

Watch out for the degree of moisture that has been left in the fruit. Some fruits are dried to a savage extent in order to give them a longer shelf life. Though soaking in alcohol or other liquid can plump them up to some extent, nothing can really compensate for shrivelled-up, over-dried fruit. So look for fruit that has a certain 'give' under the skin. Some, such as prunes, come with a moisture, or humidity, percentage on the packet. The higher the humidity, the juicier the fruit will be when reconstituted.

Avoid sulphur dioxide. This preservative is used routinely in quite large quantities to treat dried fruit, yet it is known to provoke extreme allergic reactions in some people, which can be fatal, and can also cause weakness, shortage of breath and digestive problems. It is used not only to give the fruit a longer life but to 'improve' its appearance. An unsulphured apricot is quite dark and brown in colour, while a sulphured one looks much more cosmetic, smooth and light orange in colour. Some of the sulphur dioxide can be removed by soaking and cooking but it is a real hazard for people who nibble at raw dried fruit. Most wholefood shops sell unsulphured fruit. Sulphur dioxide is not permitted in organic dried fruit.

In the **candied fruit** department, you are in the territory of lurid artificial colours. Angelica, for example, not a fruit but a plant, is often included in 'mixed candied fruits' and, even though it is quite brightly green under normal circumstances, it is commonly touched up with artificial colour. Glacé cherries are candidates for the same treatment. More natural candied fruits tend to be less vivid and paler in colour than the dyed ones, but check the ingredients listing.

When buying candied citrus, or mixed peel, check that the fruit has not had any post-harvest chemical treatment (see page 29). The bulk of candied peel is made from treated fruits. The alternative is to buy untreated fruit and candy it yourself. Armed with a decent recipe, this is a lot easier than it may seem.

Flour

Self-raising flour is low-protein (soft) wheat flour with bicarbonate of soda and tartaric acid added. These raising agents are regarded as safe. This type of flour is recommended for home baking of cakes and biscuits but not usually for bread. For more information on plain flour, see Bread.

Fruit juices and drinks

It pays to be vigilant. There is a proliferation of products that look similar but are actually radically different. Price is a useful guide to quality in this category – you get what you pay for. Chilled juices are generally better than ones that can be stored at room temperature.

In the **chilled juice** category, **freshly squeezed** juices (orange, grapefruit and so on) should be just that, and not treated in any other way. These are sold refrigerated with a short shelf life – usually two to three days. Do not assume that everything sold chilled is freshly squeezed. Other juices are also sold chilled but have been **flash pasteurised** or **heat treated** after squeezing to kill off the yeasts in the juice. These have a longer shelf life (21 days to three months) but do not taste so good, even though they are quite expensive. Some of the vitamins are killed off by the pasteurisation. The juice may also have been treated in other ways, such as clarification, filtration or putting it through a **centrifuge**. None of these treatments needs to be mentioned on the label, although they definitely affect the taste and the nutritional value of the juice. Even more confusingly, some chilled juices also combine freshly squeezed juice with a proportion of reconstituted concentrate.

Ambient juices, that is, juices sold unrefrigerated in cartons or bottles, have all been heat treated, so they do not taste or smell like freshly squeezed juice or have as many health advantages. The best are those labelled **100% unsweetened pure juice** or just **pure juice**. This means that they contain only fruit juice and no added water, colourings or preservatives. (The only exception is grape juice which may contain sulphur dioxide, a preservative worth avoiding because it can cause serious adverse reactions – see Dried and Candied Fruit). Several upmarket bottled apple juices from named apple varieties are now available and are usually of excellent quality. The flavours are clean and full of character, and each variety tastes different. They are pasteurised to give a long shelf life. This alters the flavour, so it isn't quite like freshly pressed but it comes close.

Despite the 'unsweetened' label, manufacturers can legally add up to 15 grams of sugar per litre to bring the juice up to a standard level of sweetness. This should only be done to correct the juice in overacidic batches of fruit but there are worries in the trade that it is often abused. **Sweetened fruit juice** can have 50–100 grams of sugar added to each litre.

The next quality grade down are juices **reconstituted from concentrate**. The original juice is boiled to evaporate the water, losing much of its aroma and taste in the process. This usually happens in its country of origin. Though there are regulations about the amount of pith, pulp and skin that can find their way into the juice used for concentrate, it is not clear that these are always respected. Then the concentrate is sold to producers in other countries, who dilute it with water to its original level. Over the years a series of scandals has surrounded this type of juice – too much added water, the inclusion of artificial aromas to make up for those lost, topping up with extra sugar or corn syrup to improve the flavour even though the juices are sold as unsweetened, and so on. **Frozen concentrates** are less reduced versions of commercial juice concentrates and have to be sold frozen because they do not keep as well.

Fruit nectars are usually made from fruits such as apricots and peaches, which are too pulpy to make a thin, pouring juice. These must contain a minimum of 25 per cent fruit juice but they can be diluted with water and contain up to 20 per cent added sugar. Some healthy-looking fruit nectars say 'no added sugar'; these usually contain a preponderance of tropical fruits, such as pineapple and mango, which are naturally sweet. Added vitamins go some way to compensate for those lost in processing.

Anything with the word 'drink' in it is to be avoided. **Fruit drinks** are cheap but bad value. They give you a minimum of 5 per cent fruit juice, though it may be reconstituted from concentrate. Orange juices may also be 'comminuted', which means that they contain not just the juice but the pulp and skin too. Comminuted orange juice is sometimes sold as 'whole' orange drink. This minimal amount of inferior juice is then mixed up with water, sugar, citric acid and artificial flavourings. **Fruit-flavoured drink** means that some juice has been used. Bottom of the barrel are **fruit-flavour drinks** which, despite all those pictures of luscious fruits on the packaging, do not have to contain any juice at all. They are just horrid combinations of artificial or natural colours, artificial flavours, sugar and water and have nothing whatsoever to do with fruit.

See also Soft Drinks.

Gelatine

The gelatine we use for setting mousses is extracted from animal carcasses by boiling up the skin and bones, sources of natural gelatine. The carcasses are either what is known as 'casualty animals' – they have had to be culled through accident or illness – or those whose productiveness has dropped, such as exhausted sows and old dairy cows. The latter category is particularly worrying, since gelatine could well contain the as yet unidentified 'infectious agent' that has caused BSE, or mad cow disease (see page 119). What's more, gelatine comes out of a huge melting pot of carcasses derived from many sources, so it is not easy to control the contents. This is why packets usually say 'product of several countries'. Both leaf and powdered gelatine are made in this way. Some cooks find the leaf version better to handle but it is still extracted by the same methods as the powder.

Gelatine is a pretty unsavoury way to get something as sweet and delicious as a lemon mousse to set. The more appetising alternative is agar-agar which is derived from seaweed. It is available in wholefood stores and some chemists. It sets more firmly than gelatine, so recipes need adjusting.

Honey and other sweeteners

The cheapest and most basic honey available is **blended honey**. This has been bought in from different sources and mixed to achieve a particular style. Such honey can be spotted quite easily because it is labelled 'product of several countries'. Other cheaper honeys may come from a single source – often China – but are regarded in the trade as poorer quality. Such honey is the least interesting around, and is commonly pasteurised or heat treated to postpone its natural crystallisation and thus give it a longer shelf life. Better honey comes from a specific location, a named farm or apiary, and will detail the type of flower or blossom from which it is derived. Honey sold on the basis of a country of origin, such as Mexican or Greek, followed by the name of the blossom, such as clover, may be a blend from anywhere in that country, albeit of one blossom type. As a general rule, the darker the honey, the stronger it will taste and the more aromatic it will be.

Honey in the comb has not been treated or processed in any way. Once it has been removed from the comb, honey packers heat it until it is clear and runny and strain it to remove any impurities. There are then two alternatives. The first is to put it in jars and sell it as **runny honey**. Eventually this honey will crystallise again naturally. The speed of crystallisation depends on the type of honey, with higher-dextrose honey (such as oil seed rape, usually sold as 'blossom' or in 'mixed flower') crystallising quickly and lower-dextrose honey (such as acacia) taking longer.

Some consumers don't like honey that crystallises, so **thick-set honey** can be made from the runny honey after heating by adding a little set honey to it. This speeds up the process and offers a honey that will not change in the jar after you have bought it.

Certain honeys, often Greek and German, are not strictly honey at all but what is known as **honeydew**. This is actually the excreta of aphids and other little insects that the bees have collected, as opposed to honey which the bee collects from the secretions of pollen in flowers. In certain countries honeydew sells as a premium product. It is generally darker in colour and will stay liquid in the jar. Sometimes honeydew is specified on the label, sometimes not.

Maple syrup is produced in a very labour-intensive process by evaporating sap collected patiently from the maple tree. It has a marvellous flavour. The same cannot be said of **maple-flavoured syrup** which is just cheaper corn or sugar syrup with artificial flavourings added. **Pancake syrup** is usually corn syrup with some maple syrup added. Most maple syrup is of extremely high quality and a completely natural product. A maple leaf symbol is put on such syrups and a 100 per cent pure grade A declaration. Organic maple syrups are also available in wholefood shops.

Golden syrup is made from the sap of sugar cane. **Molasses** is the syrup left over after sugar has been crystallised from sugar cane and comes in two forms, either as lighter or 'first' molasses, then black treacle or blackstrap molasses. This is the part of the sugar cane that contains the nutrients, such as vitamins and minerals.

Corn syrup is runnier than golden syrup, often used in American recipes and comes in two forms: light or dark, which has some molasses added.

See also Sugar and Sugar Substitutes.

Jams, jellies, marmalades, chutneys and relishes

One of the most puzzling things about **jams, jellies and marmalades** is how different brands with seemingly similar ingredients can all taste so different. You can deduce a certain amount by the declaration of fruit on the label, which tells you what proportion has been used: 40 grams of fruit per 100 grams is a better-than-average jam, 50 grams is better still and 70 grams is about as high as you can go before the jam turns into a compote – that is, it won't set. Generally, the higher the percentage of fruit the better, although acid fruits, such as citrus in marmalade, are usually lower. The proportion of fruit used is the simplest way to assess the quality of a jam.

However, what the percentage doesn't tell you is the quality of the fruit used. The most basic sort of **jam** is made with what is known in the trade as 'fruit crumble', which is the fruit left on the cane, tree or bush after an initial picking for the best fruit. Such fruit is less than perfect and often quite broken up. It is frozen or reduced to concentrate to sell to jam or yogurt manufacturers. These processes cause it to lose much of its freshness, flavour and colour. Better-quality jams use fruit grown for the purpose, sold direct to the manufacturer, then frozen. This type of fruit is usually very high quality. The very best jam is made with fruit that has been freshly picked and not frozen. Obviously, this is a seasonal activity and is popular only with small producers, who do not rely solely on jam for their income.

Jams, jellies and marmalades need a minimum total sugar content (including added sugar and sugar in the fruit) of about 60 per cent, to stop them going mouldy. Various other sweeteners can be substituted. An increasing number of quality jams are made with unrefined cane sugar (see Sugar), which has a better flavour than white sucrose or glucose syrup and contains a tiny amount of valuable nutrients. Fructose or fruit sugar is also thought to give a better flavour. Apple juice concentrate can be used and gives a healthy image but is still very sweet. Jams made with these types of sugars are often not as clear and brilliant as sucrose jams, appearing rather cloudy. Artificial sweeteners (see Sugar Substitutes) are often used in 'diet' and low-calorie products and have an unpleasant chemical flavour.

There are various industrial methods for making jam, most of which involve boiling the fruit to death in order to get a firm set, so the jam ends up tasting and smelling of nothing but sugar. Smaller jam manufacturers work with traditional open cauldrons or pans like giant jelly pans. Less jam is made at any one time and more care is taken in seeing that the fruit isn't overcooked. These jams tend to taste fresher and more home-made. Increasingly, manufacturers are trying to produce jams that taste of fruit by reducing the sugar content and upping the fruit. The technical problem here is that the jam doesn't keep as well, so in order to maintain their generous use-by date, a chemical preservative such as potassium sorbate is added. There are doubts about the safety of this group of preservatives (E200–213), which is suspected of causing allergic reactions, gastric irritation and problems with conception, amongst other things. Many smaller manufacturers get round the problem by having a shorter use-by date and recommending that you keep the jam in the fridge once opened.

Citric acid, which is thought to be quite safe when used in

small quantities, is often included in commercial jams to stop the colour fading and prevent the browning that occurs in some fruits such as raspberries and strawberries. It can also be used to disguise fruit of inferior quality and overcooked jam.

Pectin, a traditional gelling agent which is prepared commercially from apple cores, is often added to help the set. This is necessary for fruits that do not have enough pectin of their own, such as blueberries and cherries. The less sugar used, the more pectin becomes necessary.

A minority of poor-quality jams and fruit jellies still use artificial colourings and flavourings to disguise the pitiful quality of the miserably small amount of fruit they contain. You can spot them a mile away by their garish colours, rubbery set and artificial fruit pastille smell. Caramel is used widely to colour marmalade.

No-added-sugar jams are usually made by substituting concentrated apple juice for sugar. This often means that you get a fruitier jam but much depends on the brand. Some are very good and taste fresh and natural, while others are still surprisingly sweet and don't have a fresh-fruit taste. Most no-added-sugar jams use wholesome ingredients but it still pays to read the ingredients list carefully: certain brands use artificial sweeteners and some of the more unpleasant additives associated with cheap jams.

Careful scrutiny is required when buying **lemon curd**. Despite their twee and rustic packaging, curds are usually made with dried pasteurised egg, lemon juice concentrate, loads of sugar, phoney lemon flavouring, preservatives, emulsifiers and even colouring. A traditionally made lemon curd consisting of just fresh eggs, lemons and sugar is like gold dust.

Chutneys, relishes and other condiments are made along similar lines to jams, as they contain a lot of sugar. The best ones use top-quality fresh vegetables and dried fruits, plus good wine vinegar, while the bad ones contain a large portion of the undesirable additives mentioned above, along with cheap spirit or malt vinegar (see Vinegar), so you generally can't taste anything else.

Margarine and spreads

Margarines and spreads are widely promoted as alternatives to butter because they contain more polyunsaturated and less saturated fat. In recent years though, the health benefits of many low-fat margarines and spreads have been called into question. Most spreading margarines are made with **hydrogenated** (chemically hardened) vegetable oils and many scientists believe that this process converts the more desirable polyunsaturates into something called **transfats**, which may be every bit as harmful as saturated fat. It is thought that they delay the absorption of fatty acids and raise the levels of bad cholesterol in our blood, while some research even links them to heart disease.

This particular debate notwithstanding, what sort of product is margarine? Unlike butter, which is a natural product made simply by churning cream (see page 161) margarine is a highly processed and artificial food. It is usually made by combining water and vegetable oils, though some spreads include a proportion of butter to give a better flavour. Some margarines still include animal fat.

The oils used are generally cheap commodity oils such as palm, rapeseed, sunflower, cottonseed, safflower and grapeseed, which have been industrially refined (see Oils). Sometimes more upmarket-sounding oils are used, such as olive oil, but these have usually been industrially refined just like the commodity oils and have lost much of their taste and nutritional qualities. They are bought in from a variety of sources, many of which have blended oil from different locations.

These liquid oils are hydrogenated and then blended with water. Because fat and oil do not usually blend, emulsifiers have to be added to bind them together. The most common of these are lecithin and monoglycerine. Some spreads also use animal gelatine (see Gelatine), as well as modified starch, to give a better consistency. To add flavour and also to stabilise the spread, some whey left over from milk is added. A preservative such as

241

potassium sorbate (suspect as a mutagen amongst other things) is included to give a longer shelf life and to preserve the other additives in the spread. Not surprisingly, none of this tastes too delicious, so the flavour is 'corrected' with lactic acid, milk sugar (lactose), artificial flavourings and sometimes salt. The hue is 'improved' by the addition of colourings, usually natural ones such as beta-carotene. Artificial vitamins are often added to restore some of those lost in processing and to bring it back to the vitamin level of butter.

The worst-tasting products in this category are **low-fat and low-calorie** spreads. The only real difference between these and other margarines is that you are paying for extra water in place of fat. Otherwise, all the same objections apply.

Certain brands of spread, available mainly in wholefood shops, use healthier **cold-pressed oils** and **non-hydrogenated vegetable oil**. These usually carry a 'no hydrogenated fat' label and unless a spread has this guarantee you can assume that the liquid vegetable oils have been hydrogenated. These are usually listed as 'vegetable fat' (as opposed to oil), 'partially hydrogenated' or 'mono and di-glycerides of vegetable oil'. If you want to eat spreads, these are the ones to go for.

On the flavour front, spreads can never compare with butter, and for those who like to eat whole, unprocessed food in as natural a state as possible, this combination of fat, water and additives – hardened or otherwise – is less than appealing. If you want to cut down the saturated fat you eat, unhydrogenated spreads are one way of doing it but there are no other health benefits. Many people might prefer simply to stick to butter and just eat less of it!

Mustard

There is a marked difference between the English style of mustard and the French, or Continental, style. English-type mustards are made from **white or yellow mustard seed**, which has a blander, less aromatic flavour than the **black or brown mustard seed** used in France. (Some English mustard is a blend of both.)

English mustard often has no vinegar in it, using the chemical citric acid instead to give sharpness. English-type wet mustards usually taste hotter than Continental ones because there is no vinegar to offset or counterbalance the heat of the mustard. **Powdered mustard** tastes especially hot for the same reason.

Sugar is common in English mustards but not in their French equivalents. It is also used a lot in American mustards, where a sweeter flavour is preferred. When vinegar is used in English mustards, it is in those made in the French style but it tends to be spirit vinegar, a cheap basic item with a harsh edge and no flavour. Real French mustards are made with wine vinegar, which is a far superior product (see Vinegar).

It seems to be traditional in English mustards to add white wheatflour as a thickener, which gives a stickier, grittier effect in the mouth and less flavour. English mustards also frequently contain artificial colourings such as tartrazine, a derivative of coal tar, which provokes adverse reactions in some people.

Fewer French mustards contain colourings, but even leading brands include preservatives such as potassium metabisulphite. This belongs to a highly suspect group of additives which provoke severe reactions in some people and are possibly carcinogenic.

The best basic mustards of whatever type have very simple ingredients – water, mustard seed, vinegar and salt. Any additional ingredients should be natural items such as herbs, spices and wine, not the chemical ones mentioned above. Wholegrain mustards usually contain little in the way of unnecessary additives.

Nuts and seeds

Though we tend to think of them as a dry store item, nuts of all kinds – walnuts, hazelnuts, almonds, pine kernels, brazils, pistachios, pecan, chestnuts and so on – should really be treated like fresh food. They are quite oily and go rancid quickly when exposed to oxygen. The same applies to seeds such as sunflower and sesame, although these do stay fresh longer.

Commercial nut wholesalers get around this problem by kiln-drying the nuts, both in the shell and out, which means that they can be sold with a much longer shelf life. However, kiln-drying tends to remove much of the flavour and natural appeal of fresh nuts, which should be moist and creamy, with a mild, slightly sweet taste. Unfortunately, many dried nuts, especially walnuts, are shrivelled up, dry and bitter. Positively nasty!

Buy nut kernels and seeds pre-packed and pay attention to the use-by date. These are far too generous as a rule, so try to use them long before. Loose nuts and seeds are best avoided unless you are absolutely sure that the shop has an excellent turnover. Taste them first before you buy. With nuts, go for either whole nuts or halves, not pieces, since they are likely to be fresher. Otherwise, look for nice even-sized nuts which are not broken or sitting in nutty dust. Paler nuts (walnuts especially) usually taste fresher than dark ones. Staleness, rancidity or extreme bitterness is not acceptable – take nuts like these back. There are no bargains in the nut world, despite the disparity in prices within one nut variety. You get what you pay for.

One thing to look out for is nuts in their freshest form – just as they come off the tree. These have not been kiln-dried and are sold as fresh. Hazelnuts (also called filberts and cobnuts) and almonds still have their outer husk on, which is spiky on the former and furry and green on the latter. Walnuts, referred to as 'wet walnuts', look the same as dried, though the shells generally seem fresher and blonder in colour. These nuts are a seasonal treat and usually found only in top shops at high prices. But they are a taste worth trying, even if only once, to see what a truly fresh nut is all about. English cobnuts are available in the autumn, French and Spanish almonds may appear as early as the summer, and wet walnuts (usually French) become available from October until Christmas, depending upon the region.

Oils

Basic **cooking oil** is produced by a highly industrial process. The raw material is crushed, heated and pressed, neutralised, bleached and deodorised using chemical solvents, phosphates, alkalis and high temperatures. The goal is to produce a neutral-tasting oil that will keep well. In the process, most of the volatile aromas, which give the oil its characteristic flavour, and the nutrients (mainly vitamin E) are destroyed. These bland cooking oils are made from commodity crops such as sunflower, groundnut, corn, grapeseed, safflower and rapeseed (colza), which are bought and sold on the world market. **Vegetable oil** is just a blend of refined commodity oils. You can assume that all the cooking oil you see is produced this way, unless the label states otherwise. **Pure olive oil** is produced in a similar way, but a small proportion of better-quality virgin olive oil is added to give it colour and flavour.

    Cold-pressed oils are produced by a mechanical process. Seeds, nuts or olives are put through a hydraulic press and filtered. This is a natural method of oil extraction, which conserves the flavour and the aroma of the raw material. Less oil is extracted this way because the raw material cannot be heated, so this makes it more expensive. Cold-pressing is therefore used for high-value oils such as extra virgin olive oil and nut oils.

    Cold-pressed **seed oils**, such as sunflower and groundnut, have a distinct flavour compared with their refined equivalents and are not at all neutral. (One exception to this is refined sesame oil, which has a strong flavour because the seeds are dark-roasted first. Unroasted sesame oil, which is cold-pressed, has a definite flavour but it is not so intense.)

    Nut oils can be either cold-pressed or extracted by roasting the crushed nuts and then squeezing out the oil. Although the nuts have been heated in the latter method, and therefore don't qualify as 'cold-pressed', they are not industrially refined. In taste terms, oils from roasted nuts tend to have a more toasted, verging on acrid flavour than cold-pressed ones, but the difference is very slight.

Cold-pressed seed and nut oils, and roasted nut oils, go rancid quickly and so are best stored in the refrigerator. Cold-pressed virgin olive oil is best kept in a dark place at no more than 20°C.

VIRGIN OLIVE OIL

The legal definition of **virgin olive oil** says that it should be 'oil produced from the fruit of the olive tree, solely by mechanical or other physical means under conditions, particularly thermal conditions, that do not lead to alterations in the oil, and which has not undergone any treatment other than washing, pressing, decantation, centrifugation and filtration'. What this means effectively is that virgin olive oil cannot be 'refined' in an industrial process, while 'pure' olive oil can be.

Virgin olive oils have been extracted by a natural process which, though increasingly mechanised, observes the age-old principles of olive pressing.

Within the category of virgin olive oils that are considered fit for consumption (some are not and are called *lampante*), there are three grades. These grades relate to the acidity level of the oil which is used as an indicator of quality. **Extra virgin olive oil** must contain less than 1 gram per 100 grams, **fine virgin olive oil** less than 1.5 grams, and **semi-fine** or **ordinary virgin olive oil** less than 3 grams. In practical terms, it is increasingly only extra virgin olive oil that is sold in the UK.

Cold-pressed means that no heat has been used in the pressing process. This would release more oil but generally of a higher acidity level and therefore of lower quality. **First cold pressing** means that the oil has been obtained from the first, not subsequent pressing.

Within the extra virgin olive oil category, there is a wide price spectrum. Most cheaper extra virgin oils with familiar brand names are blends of several extra virgin oils that have been bought in – mainly from Spain and North Africa – and blended to the preferred house style. Just because an oil says 'Product of France' or 'Product of Italy', you cannot assume it was produced there, simply bottled there (see page 138). Most of this is good, workaday oil, although it is often surprisingly neutral and unaromatic in character.

Even though these are extra virgin olive oils, they are not necessarily top-quality ones. Many are bought on the world commodity market and have not been produced with any great pride or drive for quality. Growers may have allowed the olives to drop off the tree (when they are almost too ripe) rather than harvesting them by hand-picking. Others may have been stored for a while. Most are respectable but not outstanding.

Better-quality olive oils will specify either on the label or on accompanying information:

• that they are both produced and bottled by the same company, for example '*prodotto e imbottigliato*' on Italian

or

• that they are from a certain estate or region

or

• who grew them (a named grower or a local co-op).

Many of them give details of the variety of olive used, though many fine oils are blends of different olive varieties from the same estate, mixed to obtain the favoured house style. More producers are also including details of how they look after their trees, whether or not they are organic and what, if any, chemical treatments have been used in cultivation. Most extra virgin olive oils in this group are extremely fine products and command high prices. Sorting them out is a question not of good or bad but of style and preference. Like Scottish malt whiskies, it is hard to find a bad one.

A little information can be gleaned by looking at the colour of the oil. Greener oils come from olives that have been picked earlier, usually to avoid any frost. These tend to come from more northern regions – Tuscany for example – and contain more chlorophyll.

They are likely to taste greener and more peppery. More orangey-green oils have been picked later in more southern regions, where growers can afford to wait longer. The ideal time is when the olive is not fully ripe but on the turn. At this point the chlorophyll has been taken over by beta-carotene. Such oils often taste lighter, fruitier and more almondy.

Cloudy oils, some of which have a sediment, are simply oils that have not been filtered, so they have more vegetable material in them. These oils keep less well, though the use-by date is still generous – two years for example. Some people consider they have more flavour and aroma, although they may look less elegant.

Pasta

Dried pasta is a reliable and useful storecupboard item. It is usually made with durum wheat semolina, a hard wheat. Wholewheat and other flours can be used but generally produce more solid results. Dried **egg pasta** contains egg as well – usually dried pasteurised egg – and has a slightly richer flavour than other dry pasta. Dehydrated spinach or tomato powders of varying quality produce green and pink pasta respectively. This pasta is generally extruded (squeezed out) from industrial pasta machines, then oven-dried. More traditional brands of dried pasta allow the freshly made pasta to dry slowly and progressively at room temperature, which is thought to produce a better flavour. Another good sign is the use of fresh eggs. This is more expensive and time-consuming but the flavour is superior. Some brands are labelled 'fresh eggs cracked at the moment of preparation'.

Fresh pasta, either plain or stuffed, is usually made with eggs and uses softer wheat flour, which makes it easier to work. Fresh should mean just that: you should consume it on the day it is made. In theory, fresh pasta is a great treat. Made at home, or bought from a top-quality fresh pasta shop, it can be sublime. Though most mass-produced 'fresh' pasta does not reach the dizzy heights of Italy's top pasta shops, the unfilled versions – tagliatelle, spaghetti, fettuccine and so on – can be quite good and an interesting change from dried. However, most mass-produced stuffed or filled pasta is solid, leaden and conspicuously short on flavour and authentic ingredients.

A lot of commercial pasta is sold in modified-atmosphere packaging (see page 49), which has the effect of slowing down ageing and decay, thus giving the product a longer shelf life. This endows 'fresh' pasta sold in chilled counters with a counterfeit freshness in comparison with the real thing. It will also have been pasteurised to make it keep better.

Worst is **dried 'filled' pasta**, which does not need refrigerated storage. It has had various types of drastic heat treatment and frequently contains chemical preservatives and flavour enhancers.

Stuffings in commercial filled pasta tend to be pretty poor. Rubbery, tasteless ricotta, unspecified 'hard cheeses', pallid flavourings, meat of no great distinction, the usual cheap, industrial bulk fillers … all at a vastly elevated price over workaday dried pasta.

Peppercorns

Peppercorns, be they green, white or black, are all fruit of the same vine – *Piper nigrum*. **Green peppercorns** are berries that have been picked underripe and therefore green. A small proportion of green berries are either kiln-dried for use in pepper mills or preserved in brine. The rest are dried, and in the process shrink and blacken. These are what we know as **black peppercorns**. **White pepper** comes from berries picked when slightly riper. Their outer casing is removed, which makes them less hot and paler in colour. **Pink peppercorns** are the berries of a totally different shrub and have a subtle, elegant flavour.

Some **late-harvested black peppercorns** are now on sale in specialist shops. These have been allowed to ripen on the vine until they turn a reddish colour. Once harvested by hand and dried, they have a deeper, more three-dimensional flavour, with spicier overtones than standard black pepper.

Like other dried spices, pepper tends to be sold in an anonymous way so it is impossible to tell where it is from.

As with all spices, freshness is very important. Much black pepper is sold past its use-by date (which is generous to start with) or packaged in such a way that it becomes stale quickly (see Saffron, Other Spices and Dried Herbs).

Pulses

Pulses (chickpeas, kidney beans, lentils, flageolets, butter beans and so on) are a great storecupboard item in either their tinned or their dried form. Like tomatoes, they seem to can well and they lend themselves to genuine convenience with no acute flavour or texture loss.

Although dried pulses can keep for years at a time they do dry out progressively and will need increasingly longer cooking, even when presoaked. Good dried pulses should look smooth, even and not broken up. Tiny holes, or a floury dustiness in the packet or jar, suggests that the contents are too old, were badly handled in transportation or may have been infested with weevils or similar insects.

Most pulses are bought in from various sources around the world and then packed in the UK. They do not usually carry a date telling you when they were dried, since it is difficult to track the age of each consignment. Dried, new-season pulses from the El Barco de Avila region in western Spain are stocked by a few adventurous specialist food shops. They have a drying date, come from one specific source and are much fresher. This shows up in thinner skins when reconstituted and a creamier consistency.

Although they are hard to find in the UK, it is worth remembering that pulses taste at their very best when fresh. These have a particular creamy moistness and savour which you will not find in ones that have been dried, then sat around for months and years. In the UK, fresh pulses are only found at present in small market gardens growing unusual varieties of vegetables.

Ready meals or recipe dishes

However appetite-whetting the picture on the box might be, however high the price tag, however fashionable the image, ready meals *never* come up to the standard of fresh food cooked competently at home. If you are a single person or a childless couple, and short of time or low on basic cooking skills, the best ready meals make a less expensive alternative to eating out in a restaurant, and may offer a higher standard of food than you can muster. But for an entire family, ready meals work out prohibitively expensive. If you like cooking, and do so reasonably well, you'll probably find yourself disappointed by the flavour.

This is because this type of food is prepared by making vast quantities to a set recipe in an industrial kitchen, which involves assembling it, cooking it, quickly reducing the temperature by stages according to a controlled regime, then chilling it. Hence the name, cook-chill. Strictly speaking, ready meals should be called 'twice-cooked', or 'reheated', meals but not in the complimentary sense. A casserole made at home may be better on the second day but the taste of cook-chill ready meals is often not that different from canned or pressure-cooked food. The worst effects are to be tasted in chicken, which usually takes on a familiar tinned-soup, processed taste.

The concept behind ready meals is convenience, and the illusion that you can get something just as good as you would make at home but without the effort – the assurance that your dish has been made according to homely methods, just writ large. However, it is obvious from tasting even the most upmarket ready meals that taste does suffer in the process. One reason for this is the basic recipes, which are rarely authentic. These recipes must then be adapted so the technical equipment for making them can cope. They may have to contain compromise ingredients especially designed for food processing use. Though today's smart convenience meals contain none of the horrors that were found in the TV dinners of yore and which persist in the poorest, nastiest processed foods, they frequently contain items that would never appear in a home-cooked version, such as sugar, dextrose, milk powder, gelatine and modified starch.

Being disappointed is one thing, being affected by food poisoning is another. Ready meals are particularly susceptible to contamination from pathogenic bacteria such as listeria, and studies have detected this bug in a worryingly large number of them. Though bigger retailers make sure the cold chain is maintained, some strains of bacteria can survive the regulation temperature. The risk is exacerbated by two factors. First, domestic fridges rarely operate at as low a temperature as is assumed, and so bacteria-prone ready meals are often incorrectly stored. Secondly, many leading makes of microwave ovens have been shown to heat food unsatisfactorily, leaving 'cold spots' in dishes that otherwise look piping hot. In fact, there may not have been sufficient heat to kill off any pathogenic bacteria.

If you eat ready meals, buy those with ingredients that are as close as possible to the ones you would use if making the dish at home. Use them as soon as you can, and make sure you reheat them very thoroughly.

Ready-to-use sauces

Ready-to-use sauces destined for pasta, rice, fish or meat come in various shapes and forms. The most common are bottled **tomato-based sauces**. All of these are heat treated so they will keep at room temperature, and as a result never taste like a comparable sauce made at home. There are, however, various quality grades within this bracket.

The best ones are made with fresh tomatoes and will state that on the label. Some even give a breakdown such as 'prepared with 1 kilo of fresh tomatoes to make 200 grams of sauce'. Most sauces are made from either tomato pulp (described on the label as 'tomatoes') or tomato concentrate. This latter category is usually accompanied by water, which is needed to thin down the concentrate.

Tomato purée mixed with water has none of the natural thickness of well-reduced tomato sauce, so modified starch and other thickeners are frequently added, as they are to most **curry and stir-fry sauces**. Sugar is another common ingredient, often in quite a large quantity. Preservatives are often added to the cheaper ones to extend their shelf life. Vegetables, meats, herbs, spices, salt and stock bases are used as flavourings for the relatively tasteless mass, rather than as bulk ingredients. Sauces with meat in them sometimes contain undesirable flavour enhancers in the form of monosodium glutamate and yeast extract to lend a meaty effect.

When buying these sauces, it pays to read the list of ingredients carefully. Sauces made with concentrates are not likely to taste that great. Avoid ones containing ingredients you would never include in a similar recipe at home – starch, preservatives, flavour enhancers, and items such as water and sugar which appear high up the list.

Short-life pasta sauces sold chilled are generally made from more upmarket ingredients and taste fresher. But many still contain the thickeners and sugars mentioned above.

There is no reason at all for **pesto, olive and sun-dried tomato sauces** to contain preservatives, sugar, thickeners or water. The type of oil used should be specified, for example extra virgin olive oil or sunflower and so should the cheese, if included. In a pesto, for example, you should look for parmigiano reggiano or grana Padano. Descriptions such as 'hard cheese' and 'oil' do not bode well for quality.

Rice and other grains

Considering the cooked bulk they provide, even the most expensive rice is a relatively cheap item in the total cost of a meal or dish. You really get what you pay for with rice, and a few pence can be the difference between one that cooks well, smells good and has grains that stay separate, and one that turns to glue and mush. Don't be stingy.

Amongst the generally acceptable **long grain white rices**, true **basmati** and **Thai fragrant** (also known as Jasmine) rice vie for number-one place. Both guarantee fragrance and flavour and, when correctly cooked, nice, smooth, polished grains which hold their shape agreeably in the mouth. By comparison, anonymous long grain rice is pretty characterless.

In the **short grain** category, Italian risotto rice is the most satisfactory but it should be **arborio** type or, better still, **Carnaroli** or **Vialone Nano**. All three hold their shape well but the latter two are particularly elegant and produce a better 'bite'. Steer clear of anything sold as risotto rice that does not bear one of these names, as it will tend to be starchy and cook into rice pudding. **Calasparra** rice from Spain is a top-quality short grain rice with a firm round shape and performs in a similar way to proper risotto rice. **Pudding** rice is usually undistinguished short grain rice which, as its name suggests, is only really any good for one thing – pudding.

Unlike white rice, **brown rice** has not had its nutritious bran layer removed and therefore has a nuttier, more filling quality, as well as being better for you. The best varieties of brown rice are the long grain ones, sold as **Indica** or **Patna**. These cook faster and stay more separate than the stubby, short grain brown rice of the **Japonica** type, which tends to end up gummy and puddingy. Long grain varieties cost more in the UK since they are imported from outside the European Union and therefore attract duty, whereas short grain brown rice is farmed in Europe and qualifies for subsidies. If you like brown rice, it is a good idea to buy organic varieties.

Rice farming is chemical intensive and most residues will concentrate on the bran. In white rice, these are more likely to be milled off.

Par-boiled or easy-cook rice has been steam-processed. Rice treated in this way loses fewer nutrients in the milling than ordinary rice and it also tends to stay firmer when cooked, though some people think the flavour is inferior.

Wild rice is actually an aquatic grass, with a particularly earthy, nutty flavour. The quality varies, and can be judged by the final length of the cooked grain and the degree to which it holds its shape. The longer and more intact, the better. Organic wild rice tends to be of the best quality.

Red rice is a short grain rice which is a speciality from the Camargue area of France. It has a pronounced grainy-nutty flavour.

Sticky rice is meant to be that way and is destined for use in Chinese and other Southeast Asian dishes, such as steamed glutinous rice and sushi.

For other grains, such as millet, couscous, maizemeal (polenta), bulghur (cracked wheat) and quinoa, the same principles apply as when selecting grains for breadmaking (see page 193). Stoneground grains generally have a better flavour than industrial roller-milled ones, since the stones grind them less finely. They do not get warmed up as roller-milled ones do, which means they usually have more character and texture and retain more of their natural goodness. Many upmarket Italian brands of grain such as polenta are extracted by these traditional methods. Otherwise when buying grains, favouring organic ones will lower your exposure to any residues left from chemicals used in their production.

Saffron, other spices and dried herbs

Saffron filaments are the dried stigmas of the saffron crocus, prized for its yellow colouring properties and, more importantly, its complex, earthy, slightly bitter aroma. Most of the saffron in shops is Spanish. The best saffron from Spain comes from the plains around La Mancha and is usually sold as **saffron superior La Mancha**, or simply **category 1 La Mancha**. Two other grades, **Rio and Sierra**, come from different regions of Spain and are not generally considered to be of such good quality.

Some saffron, mainly Iranian, has the whiteish 'style' removed from the red filament before packing. This is known as **Corriente**, and can cost more than La Mancha saffron because the two parts are hand selected and separated. However, although the colour may be slightly stronger as a result, the flavour is not as strong since the styles contribute significantly to it.

If you can, always buy **whole saffron filaments** in preference to **powder**. Whole filaments are likely to be of the highest quality and grade and you can see what you are getting. Powders are unlikely to have been made from the pick of the crop, are more open to adulteration (though thankfully this is rare) and will oxidise more quickly and lose their aroma. Filaments, on the other hand, will keep for years in a cool, dry, dark place. If you do buy powder, usually in small sachets, make sure that it contains saffron and nothing else. It should look dark orange-red, not yellow, and may sometimes be flecked with white specks, which are the powdered remains of the styles. Check that other colourings, such as turmeric, have not been included, or worse, artificial yellow dyes, namely E102 tartrazine (*tartaracina* in Spanish). Some really poor-quality powder is to be found in Spain, usually sold as 'paella powder'. Such powders are not actively fraudulent but are often misleading, so it pays to study the label. Most powdered saffron in the UK is imported via Italy and is of a perfectly reasonable standard, though it is never as pungent as whole filaments.

No other spice has a quality-grading system like saffron. For spices in general, the most important thing is to make sure they are as fresh as possible. The best way to do this is to buy **brown spices**, such as coriander, cumin, turmeric and ginger, in the type of tins where the lid can be removed and replaced with a plastic cover. These are much better value for money than the small glass jars in which spices are commonly sold. Whole spices, such as peppercorns, are often sold in sealed plastic containers and these are fine too. It's a good idea to buy your spices from Asian stores if possible, where there is a much better turnover and therefore they are fresher.

Spices sold loose, or in twee packaging, are to be avoided. These have often been lying around for far too long and are badly oxidised. Stale spices are pretty easy to sniff out. They are usually short on aroma because they have lost many of their volatile oils in contact with air. Spices that are really old or have been incorrectly stored (too much heat, light and air) can smell quite dank, like damp dungeons or dirty dishcloths. Take them back to the shop and complain.

Dried **herbs** such as tarragon, basil, and hardier herbs such as rosemary and bay take on a different and more concentrated flavour than their fresh equivalents and cannot be substituted for fresh ones without some recipe adjustment. The most upmarket ones these days are freeze-dried, retaining more aroma and a better colour. Organic dried herbs – grown naturally without chemicals – are becoming more readily available. Certain herbs that are very fresh and green, such as parsley, chives and chervil, are not worth using dried.

Dried herbs and spices are prone to infestations and pests while in mass storage. For this reason, they used to be gassed or fumigated with ethylene oxide until this was banned on health grounds. Spices can be irradiated (see page 290) but this technology is very unpopular with consumers and so it has not been widely adopted. Now most spices are steam-cleaned – a process that entails a slight loss of colour and volatile oils but is widely regarded as safe.

See also Salt and Peppercorns.

Salt

Salt is sodium chloride and can be obtained from different sources. **Table, kitchen or cooking salt** has been extracted from underground sources, either evaporated from brine or ground up from blocks of rock salt, then purified and refined on an industrial basis. **Sea salt**, on the other hand, is produced in a much more natural manner. It is basically sun- and wind-dried, skimmed off the top of shallow seawater. Its main benefit is that the sodium and chlorine are naturally accompanied by a number of desirable trace elements and minerals that are present in sea water: magnesium, calcium, potassium, iron, manganese, zinc, copper, sulphur and cadmium. Many of these are deficient in modern diets. In standard table salt, most of these useful trace elements and minerals have been lost during refinement and purification.

Probably because of these trace elements and minerals, sea salts also have a better flavour and perfume than table salt. The finest of all is the French **fleur de sel** – the fine, light crystals that sometimes appear on the surface of the salt pans. Since sea salt is more flavoursome than table salt you can use less of it – a bonus for people who are concerned about their sodium intake.

Sea salts – especially those from the Brittany and Vendée coast of France, tend to have a greyer colour than the pure whiteness of table salt. This is how they occur in their natural state without any refining. Different sea salts have a slightly different hue and crystalline structure and the composition of trace elements and minerals varies too. When buying sea salt, favour ones that have been minimally treated to retain these. Most brands list their composition on the label. The greyer ones are superior to the white ones.

Two sorts of additive are commonly added to table salt and to the more commercial brands of sea salt. The first is an anti-caking agent, either magnesium carbonate or sodium hexacyano-ferrate, to ensure that the salt flows freely. Neither of these bestows any health advantage and there are doubts about the safety of the latter. Anyway, a couple of grains of rice in your salt cellar will stop clogging. The second is the addition of either iodine or fluoride. These trace elements are added to make up for the ones lost in purification and to give the salt a healthy image.

Low-sodium salts claim to be better for you because they substitute potassium chloride for a proportion (around two-thirds) of the sodium chloride. Though strictly speaking this does cut your sodium intake, it won't encourage you to use less in the way that good sea salt can, because it has no more flavour, other than a slight bitterness. As an additive in food, potassium chloride is known to irritate the stomach. Like regular table salt, low-sodium salt is an industrial product.

If you want to cut down your sodium intake, stick to sea salt, use less of it, and watch the hidden salt in products such as salami and biscuits.

Sauce and mousse mixes

White sauce, chilli sauce, custard sauce … dried sauce mixes sold in packets and tins are an enormous rip-off. The amount of anything even vaguely nutritious in them is tiny and they are loaded with additives to disguise the lack of decent ingredients. Standard custard powder, for example, contains modified starch (cornflour), to which sugar and artificial colourings have been added to make up for the absence of egg. Dessert mousse mixes give you all that and some added preservatives, gelling agents and emulsifiers, too. Savoury sauce mixes are big on starch, dubious flavour enhancers and an awful lot of salt. This is a category of low-grade rubbish that we can all do without.

Soft drinks

There is very little – and often nothing – that is even vaguely beneficial in soft drinks such as fizzy drinks and squashes. Colas, for example, are about 99 per cent sweetened water, with the remaining 1 per cent given over to caramel colouring, caffeine and minute traces of oils such as lime, nutmeg, cinnamon, neroli and orange. So called fruit-flavour drinks (see Fruit Juices and Drinks) contain precious little fruit juice and often none. Lemonade-type drinks are big on reformed colourings of the crudest and cheapest types and artificial flavours. Fizz is pumped in in the form of carbon dioxide.

More upmarket and expensive drinks often incorporate better-quality natural essential oils and unspecified quantities of plant extracts that are said to have health benefits, such as ginseng and guarana, and substitute naturally sweet fruit juice for other sugars. It is doubtful whether they contain enough plant extracts to give you the effect associated with the plant, which is why they do not make such claims on the label, allowing your imagination to do the rest. These drinks taste much better than the more artificial ones.

Good-quality fresh lemonade has recently become available in some supermarkets, made with just water, real lemon and sugar. It is stored in the chiller cabinets alongside freshly squeezed juices.

Diet drinks replace white sugar and other more conventional sweeteners with artificial ones (see Sugar Substitutes). These may be a health risk and they have a distinctive chemical flavour.

Sulfites – a group of highly suspect chemical preservatives – turn up frequently in soft drinks. Numbered E220–227, they have caused allergic reactions and, in certain cases, proved fatal. They are suspected carcinogens and mutagens, too. Sulfites turn up in a wide range of drinks from barley water, through sodas and mixers, to shandies.

Soups

Packet soups contain the same sort of junky additives you find in sauce and mousse mixes (see page 259) and stock cubes (see page 262). Tinned soups are slightly better quality and contain more 'real' ingredients but also large quantities of thickeners and too much salt and sugar.

More upmarket soups sold chilled with a short shelf life do not usually contain unnecessary additives and the ingredients read like ones you would use at home. These are a reasonable substitute for home-made if you are short of time but many retain that over-boiled, slightly faded, processed flavour which is reminiscent of food prepared in pressure-cookers. An improvement on tinned, but still very different from fresh, home-made soup.

Most ready-made soups are heavily salted. The quality of the stock is rarely, if ever, specified, which means that it can be recon-stituted from an industrial powder base.

Soy and other oriental sauces

When you are buying sauces for Chinese, Japanese, or Southeast Asian cooking, watch out for additives. Soy, black and yellow bean, oyster, hoisin and chilli bean sauce are all likely to include them.

Additives that crop up regularly in some versions of these prod-ucts are caramel (as a colouring), monosodium glutamate or MSG (as a flavour enhancer), yeast extract and hydrolysed vegetable protein (to lend a meaty taste), huge quantities of salt and sugar in various forms such as glucose and treacle, and modified starch. Artificial flavourings are also quite common, such as 'oyster-flavour sauce' which contains no oysters. Artificial colourings are added, too. All this stuff can give you a bad headache, leave you feeling parched and even provoke allergic reactions.

Although such ingredients seem to be ubiquitous in the widely available Westernised versions of these sauces, most good Chinese and oriental supermarkets offer a range which will include more natural, high-quality versions of the same product. Many whole-food shops also stock these, too.

As a general rule, Japanese products tend to be better and made more traditionally, so buy Japanese shoyu or tamari rather than Chinese soy. Salted black or yellow beans, for example, can also be substituted for ready-to-use sauces. If you need chilli, chop up a fresh one and so on. Your food will taste all the better for it.

Stock and 'flavour' cubes

Stock cubes are sold as an attractive, quick-fix kitchen prop. We are led to believe that we can dispense with bones and trimmings, turn hours into minutes, and produce the wholesome and appetising stocks featured on the packet: succulent meat, with steaming herb and vegetable aromas.

The reality is that the average stock cube is made up of very poor ingredients indeed, including modified starch and monosodium glutamate – a chemical flavour enhancer which causes adverse reactions in some people. This is used to give the thing some flavour. You'll find hydrogenated animal and vegetable fats (see Margarine and Spreads), which are decidedly unhealthy. The meat-flavour cubes are likely to contain hydrolised vegetable protein (HVP), an amino acid which gives a sort of meaty taste. Apart from the fact that HVP is considered a health risk and is not allowed in baby food because it may affect growth and cause tumours, its role is to disguise the lack of meat stock in the cubes. You have to go a long way down the ingredients list of most cubes before you come to anything remotely decent, such as meat, vegetables, herbs or spices. The various industrial vegetable extracts used are obviously insufficient to give the stock a flavour, so artificial flavourings, caramels and sugars frequently accompany them.

The absence of meat is probably fortuitous, since the likely candidates for stock cubing include aged 'intervention' meat from Europe's surplus meat mountains, clapped-out battery hens, exhausted milk cows and animals that have had to be put down – 'casualty' or 'fallen stock'. Their carcasses are boiled up to produce a liquid meat extract, which is then dehydrated. How yummy!

If you do not have time to make your own stock, the next best thing is the liquid stocks sold chilled in supermarkets and some specialist shops. Though these cost much more than cubes the flavour is significantly better, and they don't usually contain the nasty additives that are ubiquitous in stock cubes.

Sugar

Refined white sugar is 99.9 per cent pure sucrose and a highly processed product. Sugar can be extracted from two sources: sugar cane or sugar beet. With sugar cane there is no need to refine it, whereas sugar from beet can only be used if it is refined, since the juice is too bitter in its natural form.

In the refining process, nearly all the nutrients that normally accompany sucrose (those found in molasses) are lost or taken out, leaving calories but nothing else. The purpose of the process is to come up with bright, white granules of chemically pure sucrose, which means that chemicals and bleaching agents have to be used. **Icing sugar** (ground to a powder), **white cube sugar**, **preserving sugar** (larger crystals used for jam making) and caster sugar are all just variations on refined white sugar.

Fructose, or fruit sugar, is derived from sucrose. It is sweeter than sucrose, so you can use less of it.

Most commercial **'brown' sugars** are just refined white sugar that has been coloured by the addition of caramel or raw cane molasses. Sometimes sulphur dioxide (a highly suspect preservative; see Dried and Candied Fruit) is added. Brown sugar of this type does not have even the modest nutritional benefits associated with unrefined cane sugar.

Unrefined cane sugar (sometimes called raw cane sugar), is anything between 87 and 96 per cent sucrose and is the product of a more natural process, involving no chemical purification or bleaching. In this simpler process, the sugar cane retains more of its beneficial natural molasses. This includes other sugars, acids, B vitamins and valuable minerals, trace elements such as calcium, phosphorus, magnesium, iron, potassium, manganese and molybdenum, and phenols and other naturally occurring chemicals found in plant foods, which are thought to bestow some protection against cancer and certain other diseases.

Modern unrefined cane sugars come in various degrees of

coarseness adapted for different uses – golden, caster, demerara and so on. The darker an unrefined sugar, the more molasses has been left in. So 'golden' sugar has less and dark muscovado has more.

The natural flavour of molasses in unrefined sugars gives it a much better taste than refined white sugar and means that less can be used to obtain the same degree of sweetness. One other reason for buying unrefined cane sugar is that it comes from ex-colonial countries where entire communities (like Mauritius, Barbados and Guyana) rely on it for jobs. Most refined white sugar comes from sugar beet, which qualifies for generous European farming subsidies.

When buying brown sugar, look out for the triangular logo saying 'unrefined Mauritius cane sugar'. This is a guarantee that the sugar has not been refined and means you are not just buying coloured sucrose.

Sugar substitutes

Various intense sweeteners, or sugar substitutes, are on the market these days and widely used in a variety of foods, including yogurt, crisps, drinks, tomato sauce, lollipops, mayonnaise, biscuits, flavoured spring waters and milk drinks. All of them play to the health market, appearing in **'low-calorie'**, **'lite'**, **'diet'** and **'low-sugar'** foods. Their big claim to fame is that they are much sweeter tasting than refined white sugar (sucrose), so can achieve the same effect with much fewer calories. They also turn up in diabetic foods.

The most commonly encountered one is **Aspartame**, which is made from amino acids and is about 180 times sweeter than sugar. **Saccharin**, a derivative of petroleum, is 300 times sweeter, **Acesulfame-K**, made from sulphur and nitrogen, is 200 times sweeter. Yet another sugar substitute, **Sucralose**, is 600 times sweeter than sugar. It has not yet been approved for use.

The history of sugar substitutes began with **cyclamates**. These were derived from cyclamic acid and about 30 times sweeter than sugar. Persistent worries about their effect on human health resulted in them being banned in the UK for many years, but persistent lobbying by the food industry overcame that ban, and cyclamates may now be used legally. All the other sugar substitutes are highly controversial. Many independent scientists have doubts about their safety, either used on their own or in combination with other chemical additives such as monosodium glutamate. Such combinations turn up frequently in junk foods. There is widespread criticism of the less than open manner in which these substitutes have been tested, and the way in which so-called 'safe limits' have been arrived at.

Sugar substitutes are new and unproven. Their impact on human health is not yet known. This makes them easy to resist for those who want simple, natural food, particularly since they do not even taste very nice. They have a distinct, slightly bitter chemical flavour, almost sickeningly sweet, which is a lot less pleasant than ordinary sugar. Needless to say, they have none of the nutrients found in the better-tasting unrefined cane sugars mentioned above.

Worse flavour, more risks. Is it worth it for a few calories?

Vanilla and other flavourings

The best way to buy vanilla is as a pod. Although vanilla pods all come from the same climbing plant species, different varieties may be grown and different procedures used for harvesting. There are three main styles. The most common is **Bourbon** vanilla, which comes from Madagascar and Reunion. This is very rich, smooth, full-bodied and sweet. **Mexican** is not so rounded but is more sharp with a spicy, tobacco-like quality. **Tahiti** or **Java** vanilla tends to be more fragrant and flowery and very sweet, sometimes sickly.

When buying vanilla pods of whatever style, choose ones that are plump, shiny, moist and very aromatic. Many vanilla pods are almost desiccated when sold, and are a waste of money. They seem to keep best in glass phials.

The next best thing is **natural vanilla extract**, also called **natural vanilla essence** or **pure vanilla extract**. This is made by extracting the flavour from the beans with alcohol, then mixing it with glycerine or sugar and water. It varies in price according to the proportion of vanilla bean used. The best ones are thick and intense, usually labelled **'concentrated'**, with the inner grains from the bean suspended in the extract.

The conspicuously unsuccessful artificial substitute for natural vanilla is **vanillin**. This is synthesised chemically to copy the main flavour component in natural vanilla which is also called vanillin. However, natural vanilla also contains many more flavour components which cannot be copied – aromatic esters and oils – so artificial vanillin tastes nothing like the real thing. Many people find it positively unpleasant. Any vanilla flavouring sold as essence needs careful scrutiny. Only buy the ones listed above and avoid any that say 'vanilla flavour' or mention vanillin on the label. Avoid chocolate, confectionery, cakes and yogurts that contain vanillin. Most 'vanilla sugar' is made by adding vanillin to sugar. Some unrefined cane sugars are available containing natural vanilla extract and powdered natural vanilla pod. It is very easy to make vanilla sugar at home. Either bury a fresh vanilla pod in a jar of sugar – it will aromatise the sugar – or reuse an old, washed pod by grinding it in a food processor with some sugar. This will give a very intense vanilla sugar with 'bits' in it.

For other **flavourings** – almond, orange, lemon and so on – the same principles apply. Artificial ones are easy to spot. These taste dreadful and phoney and bear no resemblance to natural ones. They only need to be listed as 'flavouring' on the label. Some more natural-looking versions say 'with natural extract' but they usually contain artificial 'flavourings' too.

Much trickier to spot are **nature-identical flavourings**. These can vary in their make-up. Some are blends of natural essential oils which, when blended, have a similar character to the real thing. Others contain a high proportion of flavour components that have been made in a laboratory. The rule is that if more than 95 per cent of the flavouring comes from a natural source it can be labelled as natural. Nature-identical flavours have a longer shelf life than natural ones and are therefore very attractive to manufacturers. They are commonly used in scented teas such as Earl Grey, which is traditionally flavoured with bergamot oil to give a citrus flavour. If your tea label lists just 'bergamot flavouring', it is likely to be nature-identical. If it says 'natural bergamot oil', it's the real thing.

Vinegar

Vinegar is produced by allowing wine or other alcohol to sour. In so doing, they ferment and are eventually transformed into acetic acid.

Traditionally this process was a long, slow one, where the starter culture, known as a 'mother', was allowed to form naturally over time. These days, a commercial starter culture is often added to speed the whole process up – days rather than weeks.

The best **wine vinegars** (both red and white) and **champagne vinegars** are made by the traditional Orléans method. The wine, which should be of good quality to start with, is allowed to oxidise and ferment slowly so that it develops a good flavour. Then it is aged for a minimum of three months, and often for several years, in mainly oak barrels, which makes for a better taste and a rounder, smoother vinegar. **Sherry vinegar** is made along similar lines.

Vinegars produced in this way cost more than the standard commercial vinegars that have been made quickly. Increasingly, vinegar made in the traditional way is labelled with the type of wine used – Bordeaux, Chianti, Burgundy and so on. Such labels are a minimum guarantee that the vinegar has not just been made with any old wine – from the European wine lake, for example. But generally some statement on the label that the wine has been aged is more likely to be a reliable indicator of quality.

The Food We Eat

The effect of ageing vinegar is obvious when you taste properly aged **balsamic vinegar**. This is produced by evaporating juice from Trebbiano grapes, concentrating it in huge cauldrons, then ageing it progressively in casks of different types of wood – oak, chestnut, cherry, ash, mulberry and so on according to the maker's taste. The effect is a sour-sweet syrup with tremendous flavour. Purists say that balsamic vinegar should be at least 12 years old. Needless to say, this is very expensive. Commercial balsamic vinegar, which is widely available and affordable, is made by a speeded-up version of this process and is not aged in the traditional manner. It has a distinctive, sweet flavour and dark colour and is perfectly acceptable, but does not have the complexity or style of the real thing.

Cider vinegar is made from apple juice and is naturally sweeter and less acid than other vinegars.

Rice vinegar is often used in oriental cooking. It has a lighter, more dilute effect and a lower acidity than other vinegars. Japanese versions usually offer the best quality. **Malt vinegar** is made from malted barley and has a distinct flavour and a raw edge which is generally regarded as inferior to wine and other better-quality vinegars. Brown malt vinegar has simply had caramel added to it to give it colour. **Spirit vinegar** is made from alcohol distilled out of malted grain or wine. It has no virtues when it comes to cooking, though it is good for cleaning purposes. Nevertheless, it is a common cheap vinegar used in food products such as tomato ketchup.

Bottom of the barrel is what is known as **non-brewed condiment**. This is just straight acetic acid which has been prepared chemically, diluted in water and often coloured with caramel. It turns up in fish and chip shops.

Flavoured vinegars need to be chosen carefully. The cheapest ones are flavoured artificially, even though they may have a sprig of tarragon, a few raspberries, or some lemon wedges in the bottle. They tend not to taste very good. Others are flavoured with oils and extracts. These taste better than artificial ones but can be very unsubtle. The best flavoured vinegars contain only the flavouring ingredient in its natural state, such as a sprig of rosemary, and nothing else. You can make herb–flavoured vinegars at home by bruising a sprig of your chosen herb and adding it to the bottle.

Water

There are three different categories of water you can drink at home: tap water, bottled spring and mineral water, and purified (filtered) tap water. Each has its pros and cons.

Tap water is surface water that has been stored in reservoirs, pumped to filter beds where layers of sand remove fine particles and microbes, and then chlorinated to destroy any remaining bacteria. So tap water is potentially dirty water which is only clean because it has been cleaned up.

The composition of tap water is changing all the time and can include a significant proportion of water recycled through the discharge of treated sewage into rivers. Being on the surface of the land, it is vulnerable to pollution from industrial and agricultural waste.

In theory, tap water is tested thoroughly by your local water company, and official sources say that 99 per cent of tap water in the UK meets European standards. However, there are enough incidents of water contamination (often with bacteria that survive chlorination) to suggest that this figure is misleading. Environmentalists say that water purity statistics are massaged by averaging out results for 57 different types of test. This hides the fact that in a certain region at a given time water may not reach the desirable standard.

You can find out whether your water complies with legal standards either by looking at the public register held at the offices of your water supplier or by writing to ask for information to be sent. Ask for the information to show the maximum permitted levels of various substances so that you can make a comparison.

If you cannot understand it, ask your local environmental health department or Friends of the Earth for help.

Glass for glass, bottled waters cost about a thousand times more than tap water. **Bottled spring and mineral waters** are what is known as 'ground waters', which means they started out as rain which seeped through rocks and collected in underground pools beneath the earth's surface. The water can bubble up to the surface through a fault in the rocks and form a spring or it can be pumped up by drilling a bore hole. Such waters can simply be labelled **spring water**. This title can be used on almost any water that bubbles up from the ground and meets very minimum bacterial standards. **Natural mineral waters**, on the other hand, have to conform to tighter regulations.

Unlike tap water, natural mineral waters have to come from 'a naturally protected source of constant composition' and must be 'free from all traces of pollution' without the need for any disinfection or purification. The theory is that the journey of the rain through the rocks helps to purify it by filtering out the organic material that bacteria need to live on, and so they are purer than tap water. Unlike tap water, mineral water should be naturally clean. This is why most mineral waters come from relatively unpolluted areas, quiet hills and valleys free from industrial and farming pollution and so on.

In practice, a lot depends on the specific source. Some mineral waters may be only a matter of weeks old when they are bottled, because they come from shallow underground sources. Others contain water that fell as rain hundreds of years ago.

Rare incidents of contamination have occurred in mineral waters, usually introduced during the bottling process.

Most sparkling waters have had carbon dioxide pumped into them. Very few are sparkling to start with, and only these can be labelled **natural sparkling water**. Such waters are generally less fizzy than those with carbon dioxide added.

Some health benefits are claimed for mineral waters because they contain higher quantities of minerals such as calcium, which the body needs to function. The mineral composition of different waters varies, and certain waters that are heavily mineralised are not recommended for certain groups, such as babies and children, old people, and anyone who is following a low-sodium diet. These waters have a strong salty taste.

Mineral waters considered suitable for those on low-sodium diets contain not more than 20 milligrams of sodium per litre. Anything between 20 and 200 mg is regarded as moderate sodium, while anything above that is high-sodium water. People who have been advised by their doctor to cut down on calcium should look for a mineral water with no more than 150 mg calcium per litre.

If you buy bottled water, choose glass rather than plastic bottles. Some scientists think that bacteria multiply faster in plastic, and anyway, glass bottles are easier to recycle. Refrigerate the water after opening and drink it up quickly – preferably that day. Bottled water is prone to contamination from food poisoning bacteria. The longer you leave the water opened but not drunk, the more chance there is of these bacteria increasing.

Purified tap water is water that has been filtered at home, although it is now on sale in some pubs and restaurants. It has two advantages over mineral and spring waters. First, it is much cheaper. Second, a good filter system can adjust any undesirably high levels of minerals in line with modern medical thinking.

Depending on the system's degree of sophistication, filtering will remove some or all of any worrying contamination that might remain in water after treatment by the local water company.

Water filters range from simple and relatively cheap jug systems to complex, multi-stage products costing hundreds of pounds. So when you buy a filter it is important to be clear on exactly what it is designed to do.

Most cheap filters only remove the chlorine and any particles or 'bits' from the water. More expensive ones use ultra-violet light, ion exchange, and a number of different ceramic earth and carbon filters. In laboratory tests, the most advanced filtration systems have been shown to remove 99 per cent of bacteria, pesticides, industrial chemicals and heavy metals.

If you have a filter, make sure you change the cartridges regularly according to the manufacturer's instructions. Dirty filters can contaminate incoming water. Bigger, more expensive systems usually come with a maintenance contract.

Although purified tap water can be demonstrably fresh and free from pollutants, the fact remains that it has been through two major purification treatments to achieve this. Natural mineral water, on the other hand, may match this standard without any treatment whatsoever.

THE BIGGER PICTURE –
Some issues to think about

Chemical-dependent farming and the organic alternative

Most of the food in our shops is produced by what are known as 'conventional' methods. That description is a bit of a misnomer, since current 'conventional' farming techniques have been dominant only for the last 50 years – a drop in the ocean of global food production since history began.

A clearer description might be 'chemical-assisted' or 'chemical-dependent' farming. The reason most food is not labelled this way is that growers and retailers think it might scare the public unnecessarily. This sort of logic has allowed chemically produced food to be seen as normal while organic farming is seen as out on a limb – despite the fact that even in its most modern forms, organic production has far stronger links with tried-and-tested farming methods, developed over time and with detailed human experience.

Chemical-dependent farming represents a relatively new experiment in our approach to agriculture and the environment. How this chapter in the history of food production will end up is anybody's guess.

Chemical-dependent agriculture

This is based on the idea that it is impossible to achieve the necessary yields to feed the world, provide food of the standard required by the modern consumer, or control pests, weeds and disease, without using chemicals. When food production is geared up to quantity in this way, farming must necessarily become big business. The traditional self-sufficient mixed farm, which rotated a range of crops and integrated that with rearing animals, becomes an 'uneconomic' way to produce food. It has therefore given way to large-scale, intensive farming.

Intensive farms open up the possibility of much higher yields – producing more food faster in one place. However, they are also much more vulnerable to pests and disease because they have moved away from the natural ecosystem, which protected the small farm through its mix of crops and activities. This means that pesticides become necessary.

Soil that has been intensively farmed becomes exhausted and less fertile than it would be if the traditional rotation of crops and resting of fields were observed. It is depleted of the natural minerals and trace elements required to grow nutritious food, and chemical fertilisers are required to give it a boost.

THE RISKS OF CHEMICAL FARMING TO HUMAN HEALTH AND THE ENVIRONMENT

There are over 400 chemicals approved for use on crops in the UK. All of these are toxic to a greater or lesser degree. There is no disputing that humans can become seriously ill when overexposed to them, nor that they have the capacity to upset the delicate ecological balance of our land and waterways for a substantial period of time. In other words, we are playing with fire.

Advocates of chemical farming assure consumers that we have nothing to fear from the 'responsible' use of chemicals, and that it is only the odd rogue farmer who misuses them. The argument goes that the application of agrichemicals is carefully monitored, that such chemicals are thoroughly tested, and that there is a system of spot checks to ensure that pesticide residues do not go above certain 'safe' limits (maximum residue limits, or MRLs). Nevertheless, in 1995 the Ministry of Agriculture, Food and

Fisheries (MAFF) was forced to issue health warnings on carrots grown in the UK after unexpectedly high residues were found. These residues come from highly toxic organophosphate pesticides used to control carrot fly, an endemic pest that seems immune to even the strongest treatments. Even where MRLs seem acceptable they are based on the notion that pesticides are safe until proven harmful, which means that we may only be wise after the event. The history of agrichemicals is littered with toxic substances that were considered safe and then consequently withdrawn when they were shown to be dangerous, long after doubts had been raised about their safety.

It is worth remembering that many agrichemicals are potential human carcinogens, and that there is no such thing as a harmless level of a carcinogen. Others are teratogenic (affecting unborn children) or are mutagenic.

Both the acute and chronic effects of pesticides in our food chain may not be proven either singly or cumulatively, until many decades after exposure. A significant number of agrichemicals are long-persistence chemicals, which means they linger on in the environment and the food chain long after they are used. Particular worries relate to children, who are not taken into account when it comes to calculating risks because these are worked out on the basis of an average for the whole population. According to the US National Academy of Sciences, children may be exposed to two or three times the adult equivalent of chemical residues, at a time when their immature bodies are less able to cope with them.

As far as the environment is concerned, agrichemicals are proving to be a disaster. This expresses itself in the pollution of rivers and lochs by toxic effluent from aquaculture (fish farming) and agriculture, the loss of wildlife and natural habitat, and an abnormally neat and tidy landscape dominated by intensively farmed swathes of land while previously extensively farmed land lies fallow.

The contribution of agrichemicals to our food choices is also dubious. Chemical-dependent farming encourages quantity of production, not quality. Today's large European food surpluses are testimony to chemical-farming methods. The visually perfect, blemish-free produce we see all round us is only made possible by the use of chemicals. These days, a growing number of consumers are looking for more wholesome, varied and nutritious food, not larger quantities of the same, standardised, calibrated harvest.

YOU CANNOT WASH OFF AGRICHEMICALS

You can always pick a slug off your lettuce or rinse the leaves to remove greenfly but unfortunately, you cannot buy 'conventionally' produced food with an opt-out clause – the chemicals are an integral part of the deal. By removing the rind from fruit and vegetables, you will be able to avoid any post-harvest chemicals on it. However, at the same time you are discarding the part containing most of the valuable fibre and nutrients that keep us healthy.

Other agrichemicals are 'systemic' – in other words, they are in the cell structure of the fruit or vegetable. For example, over 60 chemicals are permitted for use in apple growing in the UK for pest, weed or disease control, and that's not counting fertilisers. A substantial number of these are systemic. In theory, they should not be detectable in mature produce, since they are meant to be used well before harvest so that they 'disappear' before we eat them.

The occasional insights we get behind the scenes of agrichemical use suggest that we should treat these assurances with a certain cynicism. In 1994, for instance, a government spot check on British winter lettuces grown under glass (see page 30) revealed that more than a quarter of them were contaminated with illegal, or excessive, levels of pesticides.

There is some comfort in the fact that the major supermarket chains are aware of the problem and including stricter specifications on chemical use in their contracts with suppliers – more frequent testing, more spot checks and so on. But this increased vigilance is still based on the idea that there are 'safe' levels, and that a chemical is safe until proven otherwise.

Organic farming

Organic farming is often described as 'farming without chemicals'. It is true that organic farmers do not use agrichemicals but there is a lot more to it than that. Organics is a natural farming method which aims to harness natural biological processes in soil, plants and animals in order to produce healthy, wholesome food. The end goal is optimum quantities of high-quality food, not maximum output.

Unlike chemical-dependent farming, organic farming starts with the quality of soil and its fertility. Much effort is put into keeping the soil in good condition because healthy soil produces healthy food. Chemical-dependent farmers may grow the same crop in exactly the same place year after year. Organic farmers, on the other hand, combine crop rotation with careful selection of plant varieties appropriate to local conditions in order to achieve a good harvest. There is a real cost to this technique as the land is rested and therefore produces no immediate income. This is the principal reason organic food is often more expensive.

The basic idea is that healthy crops produced in this way will not need any artificial fertilisers or pest-control methods. Instead, the plants will have been fertilised via the natural richness of the soil and farmyard compost and manure. Since the crops are more vigorous and strong, they will be less susceptible to pests and disease. Any damage should be controlled by natural methods – the ecosystem of the organic farm means there will be beneficial predatory insects in the surrounding habitat to control those that are less welcome!

THE BENEFITS OF ORGANIC FARMING FOR HUMAN HEALTH, ANIMAL WELFARE AND THE ENVIRONMENT

If you are concerned about agrichemicals, buying organic food is an obvious way to avoid them. Because agrichemicals are so persistent in our environment and food chain, it is impossible to say that no organic food will contain any agrichemicals whatsoever. But there is no doubt that in most organic produce, levels will be minuscule or non-existent. That means that you are limiting your exposure to toxic substances.

There is also some evidence to suggest that organic food may be richer in natural health-giving vitamins and trace elements. Several different pieces of research comparing organic and 'conventional' produce have found that the organic foods contained higher levels of certain vitamins (such as vitamin C) and trace elements (such as iron and magnesium).

This may be partly because organic crops take longer to grow, so they contain more dry matter and less water, therefore more nutrients. Furthermore, crops grown in fertile soil take up a better and more balanced nutrient supply from it. Chemical fertilisers can cause elements such as calcium and magnesium to be so diluted in the soil that they are not taken up as efficiently by the plant.

Research in Denmark also suggests that organic food can have a beneficial effect on male fertility. In a survey carried out in 1994 by the Department of Occupational Medicine in Arhus, Denmark, men who ate organic food were found to have twice the sperm count of men who did not. Many researchers now think that pesticides and other toxins in the environment are responsible for a decline in male fertility over the last 50 years.

When it comes to animal welfare there is no doubt that organic standards are the most comprehensive and coherent in operation. The growing trend towards vegetarianism notwithstanding, many people would still like to eat meat and animal products if they could be sure that they were produced without cruelty. Although various other welfare standards exist, most of these are partial and promise far more than they deliver. For the growing number of consumers who feel concerned about the conditions of intensive livestock, organic meat, milk and eggs offer an impressive guarantee that the animals have been well looked after. More details on organic welfare standards are included in the appropriate sections of this book.

The environmental benefits of organic food are obvious. 'Conventional' farming is one of the biggest culprits when it comes to pollution of our waterways and our land. Agri-chemicals have had a very negative impact on wildlife, natural habitat and, indeed, the whole look of our countryside. Organic farming, on the other hand, combines sensible, sustainable stewardship of the land with the supply of high-quality, nutritious food.

THE COST OF ORGANIC FOOD

The biggest stumbling block for most consumers when it comes to organic food is price. It is possible for organic foods in season to cost the same as conventional ones. On imported produce, however, the disparity can be shocking, since organic foods do not benefit from the same economies of scale as conventional imports.

The disparity in price between organic and 'conventional' produce is reducing rapidly as more consumers buy organic. However, 'conventional' produce is cheaper largely because it is heavily subsidised by the Common Agricultural Policy (CAP). The price we pay does not take into account the hidden costs of this system for both human health and the environment – such as cleaning nitrate pollution out of drinking water.

The tantalising thing is that the price of organic food could tumble, and be affordable to everyone, if the CAP was reformed.

Reform is certainly on the agenda but the shape this will take is still undecided. There is considerable pressure from some quarters for environmental objectives to be given more priority when deciding on subsidies. At present, agrichemical farming is heavily subsidised by ratepayers, largely as a result of political decisions taken in Brussels and Whitehall. A further reform of the CAP to favour extensive farming could change the economics of organic food production overnight. In addition, the price of organic food is likely to fall as more people demand it, thus opening up greater economies of scale.

For such a change to happen, it is down to consumers to force the question of natural, healthy food production high up the political agenda. The seed is there, and by favouring organic food wherever possible, consumer demand can see that it germinates.

As a practical measure, the surest route to finding organic food at a reasonable price is to go direct to local producers, many of whom now operate farm-gate shops or even home-delivery schemes. With this shortened food chain, organic produce can work out cheaper than equivalent foods in shops and supermarkets. There are usually special offers on organic foods in supermarkets, making them more or less the same price as their conventional equivalents.

HALFWAY-HOUSE AGRICULTURE

Consumer concern over agrichemicals has prompted some farmers and retailers to rethink production methods. This has resulted in an approach called variously 'environmentally conscious cultivation', Integrated Crop Management (ICM) and Integrated Pest Management (IPM).

These are essentially halfway houses between chemical-dependent and organic farming. The idea is that farmers are encouraged to cut down on pesticides and use natural techniques where possible. In the first instance, it sounds very like organic farming. Emphasis is put on choosing crops that are suitable for particular soils and locations, selecting varieties with good pest resistance, reverting to traditional crop rotations, and recycling all waste materials as compost to reduce the need for fertilisers.

Growers are encouraged to use beneficial pests, such as the tiny wasp encarsia formosa, to control predators such as whitefly. Farmers can form groups to invest in hi-tech, sensitive forecasting systems, which will warn them of likely weather hazards and pest problems and allow action in the nick of time. When it comes to pesticides, the theory is that all routine, preventative spraying is rejected in favour of smaller applications and more precisely targeted formulations.

At best, these halfway-house approaches represent an honest attempt to reduce the more obvious excesses of chemical-dependent farming. At worst, they are little more than a public relations exercise to present the acceptable face of chemical-dependent farming to a doubting public.

The first problem is that, if all else fails, IPM and ICM growers can still resort to pesticides and sprays. Schemes such as the Dutch 'butterfly' one prohibit chemical pesticides but they still permit the use of chemical fertilisers and other chemical inputs. A detailed study of the National Farmers Union ICM protocol for cauliflower alone has shown that 93 chemical formulations are still permitted, 90 per cent of these being 'broad-spectrum' treatments that affect everything else in sight!

The second shortcoming is that because these schemes are partial (not fully organic) they work only under limited circumstances – usually greenhouse crops. IPM and ICM are not really applicable to crops grown in fields, although claims are made that they can be, because farmers cannot fully control the environment around them. So IPM and ICM techniques tend to be applied only to glasshouse growing, where production is much more forced than natural to start with (see page 30).

Finally, from the consumer's point of view, the proliferation of systems along these lines is extremely confusing. One scheme might permit something, another might not, since, unlike organic farming, there is no independent body regulating standards for such schemes.

All that halfway-house labels guarantee is that, in some respect, the product has been more naturally produced than it was before. In the context of crops technically induced in hi-tech greenhouses or pesticide-packed fields, that does not amount to much of a guarantee.

DIFFERENTIATING 'NATURAL' LABELS

'Natural' is one of the most abused words in the English language, particularly when it comes to food. These days, shoppers are faced with an ever-growing range of labels on food packaging all making vaguely similar, but subtly different, claims about pesticide reduction, natural methods and so on.

When you buy food without any information about how it has been produced, you can assume that it has been grown with the aid of chemicals.

Own-brand 'natural' labels that claim to be better or greener than standard produce (halfway houses) need to be treated with care. They may be an improvement but the question is, on what?

Organic labels can be trusted provided they bear the logo of a certifying body. This means that the production method has been independently verified by a recognised organic body which is prepared to guarantee that the product really is organic.

Certifying bodies in the UK include:
- The Soil Association
- British Organic Farmers and Growers
- The Bio-Dynamic Agriculture Association (Demeter and Bio-Dyn logos)
- Scottish Organic Producers Association
- The UK Register of Organic Food (UKROFS).

All of these are government monitored and subject to independent checks and controls. There are many more organic certifying organisations around the world.

Unlike the halfway-house alternatives, organic agriculture is the only system whose rules are the same worldwide and which is transparent, open to scrutiny and legally enforced.

Genetically Engineered Foods

How does this menu grab you? The meat eaters amongst you could kick off with smoked trout fillets with human growth hormone gene, followed by roasted chicken with bovine growth hormone gene. Don't worry, the vegetarians aren't left out. We've got a lovely tomato and flounder fish gene salad, and a scrummy baked potato with scorpion gene for the main course. You will all enjoy that juicy melon with virus gene for pudding, or what about a nice plate of rice pudding made with pea gene? Think it's a joke? Far from it. These are just a few of the 3,000 or so genetically altered or 'transgenic' foods that have to date been tested worldwide. Slowly but surely they are making their way to a shelf near you.

Throughout history, special breeds or strains of crops and animals have been developed. The Aberdeen Angus, for example, was developed to produce beef with excellent eating qualities. Plant breeders have cross-bred strains of potato to produce certain desirable characteristics, such as good keeping and eating qualities.

Now genetic engineering has become the new way to 'improve' our food. Unlike traditional breeding, this approach permits scientists to move genetic material – DNA – from one living organism to another, irrespective of the species barrier. While scientists once bred wheat with wheat and corn with corn to achieve characteristics such as resistance to pests, now they can take genes from anywhere.

With this new freedom, the genetic engineer can introduce human genes into animal ones, fish genes into plant ones and so on. In the future these 'transgenic' foods may contain genes from hundreds of unrelated species of animals, insects, plants and bacteria.

There are, of course, many grave reservations about transgenic foods and these need widespread public debate. What gives the scientist the right to play God and mess around with self-regulating Nature? These constructions of disparate genetic material have never before been part of the food chain and no one really knows how they will affect it. Genetically engineered tomatoes, for example, have been altered to be resistant to an antibiotic called kanamycin. The scientists responsible say that this is acceptable because the resistance will be destroyed when cooked and it will only be used for cooked products. But what if children steal some tomatoes from a field and eat them raw? Might they become resistant to this antibiotic too? A whole new range of toxins and allergens that we cannot anticipate could be produced in new sources as a result of genetic engineering. There is not even any agreement about how transgenic foods ought to be tested. Many field tests are being carried out only in Latin American or African countries, where regulatory standards and environmental controls are lax. Having been tested in conditions that would never be permitted in the USA or Europe, these foods are then released on to the market there.

Potential dangers apart, where are the clear benefits to the consumer and society? A few years back, genetic engineering was being touted as the new technology which would decrease pesticide-dependency in farming. Yet 66 per cent of tests carried out on transgenic plants between 1986 and 1992 are now known to be concerned with making them 'herbicide-tolerant'. Put simply, they are being designed to be used along with pesticides – not to replace them.

Since transgenic foods are such a major point of departure it might seem only logical that they should be labelled as such. But the large transnational companies who dominate gene research (biotechnology) think that a 'Produced with the aid of genetic technology' or similarly worded label might put consumers off. They suspect, quite correctly, that many consumers have grave reservations about transgenic foods – ethical, religious, moral, environmental. So they have argued that there is nothing to fear because transgenic foods are just a harmless extension of traditional 'improving' techniques. No need to bother the shopper with unnecessary information then, is there?

As this book goes to press, it is not clear whether transgenic foods will need to be labelled as such. Large cheese manufacturers are already using chymosin, the genetically engineered rennet substitute, to make vegetarian cheese (see page 182). The next three likely to become available are tomato paste, which could be used in pizza toppings, pasta sauces and baked beans; vegetable oil (from genetically altered oilseed rape); and products containing genetically altered soya beans. Because these may be only one ingredient in the finished product, they may not need to be declared on the label. As things stand, that bottle of tomato ketchup, that vegetarian Cheddar or that bottle of vegetable oil may be the product of genetic engineering and you could well be the last to know about it.

Sooner or later, some form of legal labelling for transgenic foods will have to be put in place but it may well be minimal. The industry would prefer to label only foods that still contain the genetically modified organism (GMO), such as a raw or cooked tomato. Foods produced with the aid of genetically engineered products, such as a vegetarian cheese produced with chymosin, would not have to be labelled because they do not contain the actual GMO. Foods refined from genetically altered plants, such as sugar from altered sugar beet, would not need labelling either. Another suggestion is that transgenic food would only be labelled if it 'differs substantially from its traditional counterpart'. Yet the difference between the two might be extremely difficult to delineate.

In the meantime, there is one course of action for the concerned consumer. Write to your supermarket and ask it to guarantee that any transgenic food it sells will be labelled clearly as such, *including those that do not contain a GMO but may have used genetically engineered material at some point in their production process.*

Food Irradiation

Food irradiation is a controversial technology which consists of exposing food to high doses of radiation. Performed correctly, it should not make food measurably radioactive but it does bring about chemical changes. It extends the shelf life and acts as a preservative, while also killing some harmful bacteria and any insects present or breeding in the food (weevils and so on).

A few years ago irradiation was being widely promoted as the technology that was going to solve all our food safety problems – destroying salmonella in chicken and so on. However, it has effectively been stopped in its tracks by the strength of public opinion. In the UK, although it is now legal to sell irradiated food, consumer resistance means that any manufacturers who might have been tempted to use it have been scared off.

Dried herbs and spices are the only category of food that looked as though it might be irradiated. However, all the large spice companies have refused to use the technique and thus tarnish their good names by association with what is widely seen as very dubious technology. All supermarkets and major food retailers have gone on record as saying that they see no use for the technology at the present time, although Sainsbury qualifies that by adding that it is keeping an 'open mind' on the question. The British army, HM Prisons and many local authorities have rejected the use of food irradiation in their catering.

The objections to irradiation are numerous. There are concerns over the safety of the process itself, based on research done on animals which produced serious adverse effects. Vitamin loss in irradiated food can be up to 90 per cent more than in untreated food. Many hygiene and catering professionals fear that irradiation could be used to disguise food that is unfit for human consumption, being neither fresh nor clean. There are major doubts relating to irradiation's ability to deal with food-poisoning bacteria. Although it can kill off some harmful bacteria, it cannot destroy all types, such as the very common listeria found in some cooked meats, soft cheeses and ready meals. It does, however, kill off lots of beneficial bacteria which would normally compete with the harmful ones and check their progress.

You are not likely to see irradiated food for sale in the UK, but if you did it would need to have a label which stated 'irradiated' or 'treated with ionising radiation'. This labelling requirement does not apply, however, to foods where the irradiated item accounts for less than 25 per cent of the ingredient total, or to food sold in restaurants or other catering establishments. Your vegeburger or spicy sausage could be flavoured with irradiated spices and you wouldn't know about it. There are also fears that irradiated food may be imported from other countries unlabelled.

For some years, the lack of tests to determine whether foods had been irradiated or not made it difficult to deter fraudulent irradiation. These tests are now coming on stream, although they are costly to do. A few spot checks to date have found irradiated food – mainly imported spices – on sale in shops but not labelled as such.

Useful Suppliers

For information on where to buy nutritious organic food, contact the **Soil Association**. Their regularly updated *Directory of Organic Farm Shops and Box Schemes* (boxes of organic produce delivered to your door) tells you where you can buy fresh organic produce direct from the producer.

Also available are five handy *Regional Guides* listing retail outlets that stock organic food. Choose from Scotland, Wales, North of England, West Country, and South and East. Each guide also contains details of buying organic food by mail order. Each of these publications costs £2.50 (please add 50p per item for postage and packing).

The Soil Association has been promoting organic farming for over 50 years. You can become a member and receive the Association's journal, *Living Earth*, which will keep you updated on organics and food-quality issues.

For more information on membership, or if you wish to buy one of the publications mentioned, please write to the Soil Association, 86 Colston Street, Bristol BS1 5BB. Tel: 01179 290661; fax: 01179 252504.

The Fresh Food Company operates a nationwide home delivery service of organic fruit and vegetable boxes and organic meat boxes. The food all conforms to Soil Association standards for production and animal welfare. The Fresh Food Company also delivers boxes of Cornish fish, specially selected, prepared, packed on ice and sent to you within hours of landing to ensure absolute freshness.

There is a range of different boxes and prices – *For children, Prime catch, Econocatch*, and so on. You can request anything from a one-off sample to monthly, fortnightly, to weekly boxes. Payment by credit card is accepted. All deliveries are made on Thursdays.

For more information contact The Fresh Food Company, 326 Portobello Road, London W10 5RU. Tel: 0181 969 0351; fax: 0181 964 8050.

Heal Farm produces meat from rare and traditional breeds of animals to very high welfare standards. It delivers mail order and accepts credit cards. For a catalogue and price list contact Heal Farm, Kings Nympton, Umberleigh, Devon EX37 9TB. Tel: 01769 574341; fax: 01769 572839.

Neal's Yard Dairy has the best selection of British and Irish on-farm cheeses in the country, and produces a regular cheese list and newsletter. It delivers mail order and accepts credit cards. For a cheese and price list contact Neal's Yard Dairy, 17 Shorts Gardens, Covent Garden, London WC2H 9AT. Tel: 0171 379 7646; fax: 0171 240 2442.

For more information about high-quality food from small producers, I recommend buying a copy of Henrietta Green's *Food Lovers' Guide to Britain* (BBC Books).

Index

The Food We Eat